The Boudoir Bible *brings the search for a healthy body,*
soul, and spirit to sexy, vibrant life.
— Elle Macpherson

Seductive wisdom requires cultivation and knowledge.
Betony Vernon's Boudoir Bible *can elevate even the most love-savvy to the status*
of Erotic Maestra or Maestro!
— Dita von Teese

The Boudoir Bible *contains everything my mother didn't know*
about sex (and if she did would have changed the subject). Every man who digs
women should read this—not to mention the obvious beneficiaries.
— Glenn O'Brien

Betony understands that sex is the center of the greater whole.
She has committed herself to exploring it, and she is right—the important thing
is to dig straight down to the core. White is the symbol of purity, but as the sum
of all colors, it can be seen as the addition of experience. On the other hand,
black, the absence of color, is pure. Betony instinctively always chose black.
— Philippe Starck

In the age of fashion and art, Betony Vernon reminds us that
true luxury is not something you can buy, but something we give to each other.
By revealing the secrets of the Sexual Ceremony, she turns fetish,
perversion, and kink into an intimate science and joyful self-expression.
— Olivier Zahm

Betony Vernon—protean, legendary, and above all, woman—
has the imagination and the courage to bring back to sex, and to the heart,
the centrality they should have.
— Francesco Clemente

The Boudoir Bible *is an essential tome for anyone looking*
to have a lifelong, deeply satisfying love life. You won't just read this book,
you will experience it.
— Aimee Mullins

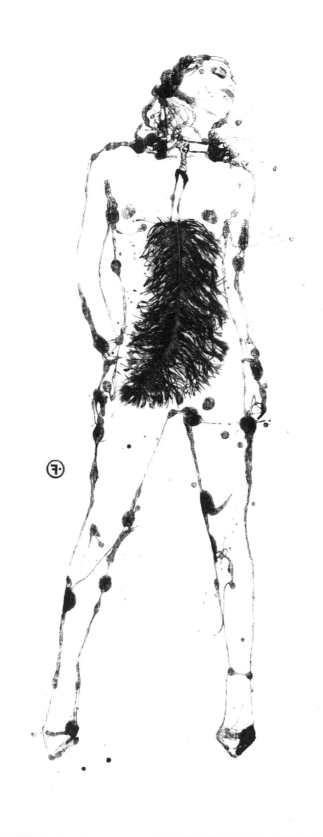

The
BOUDOIR
BIBLE

THE UNINHIBITED

SEX GUIDE

for

TODAY

by

BETONY VERNON

with illustrations by

FRANÇOIS BERTHOUD

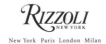

RIZZOLI
NEW YORK

New York Paris London Milan

CONTENTS

—————o—————

FOR
MY MOTHER AND FATHER,
WHO MADE MY EXTRAORDINARY LIFE
POSSIBLE.

FOREWORD

———o———

DEEP SEXUAL SATISFACTION is the foundation for enduring and meaningful intimate relationships. Whatever their sexual orientation, individuals who
enjoy more liberated, informed, and gratifying
sex lives are also known to live healthier, happier,
and more satisfying lives in general. My mission
is to empower women and men to enjoy and share
greater pleasure.

We live in a sexually charged atmosphere in
which the powers of sex and seduction are used
by mass media to generate corporate profit for
everything from pornography to an infinity of
unrelated commodities. But nowhere within this
incessant flux is the promotion of sexual well-
being and satisfaction integral to a happy and
harmonious existence.

In such a climate, sexual ignorance can only
thrive. In fact, current statistics reveal that the
needs and desires of sexually mature adults are
being fulfilled merely on a primal level. Sexual
dissatisfaction is the primary motivation that
leads couples to separate and seek divorce. This
frustrating and often debilitating condition also
helps explain why so many individuals are unable
to create enduring intimate bonds.

What ultimately keeps us from experiencing
the satisfaction that we desire and merit?

For nearly two decades I have worked as a consultant for couples and individuals on a quest to answer this vital question, which has as many answers as the number of men and women who ask it. I am not a doctor, and I don't consider those who seek my assistance as "patients." They are life-loving individuals who put their fears aside in order to seek out and attain the sexual understanding, satisfaction, and well-being that is rightfully theirs. Their trust in me and in my method, which evolves with them, gives me the rare opportunity to explore the sexual realm beyond the confines of my own personal experience. From this work I gleaned the insight that the primary culprit behind sexual disappointment is no longer the taboo against sex itself, but rather a taboo against pleasure.

Seeking pleasure is part of human nature: ultrasounds reveal that from the sixteenth week of gestation, fetuses caress their newly formed, fully differentiated genitals. Even before a child reaches the age of three, his or her sexual identity begins to take shape with the discovery of the anus and the genitals. Unfortunately, this innocent exploration does not last long—by the time we reach sexual maturity, most of us have learned to repress rather than embrace our sexuality.

The primary goal of *The Boudoir Bible* is to dismantle the pleasure taboo, helping lovers recognize pleasure-inhibiting myths, uproot misconceptions, reverse the negative consequences of social conditioning, and take full responsibility for their sexual satisfaction. To this end, *The Boudoir Bible* was not conceived as a guide in the classic sense of the term, but rather as a catalyst for sexual growth. Yet it is also chock-full of tips and instructions to help lovers cultivate sexual health and happiness. As we develop and refine our sexual skills, we begin to expand our capacity for pleasure to greater, more mutually satisfying degrees. As we unlearn pleasure-inhibiting behavioral patterns, our sexual horizons expand, and the true essence of our sexual personae may finally be unveiled.

Being that our sexual health and satisfaction are not only the result *of* but also the foundation *for* more harmonious interrelations, sexual knowledge and understanding should be the birthright of every adult. No matter what race, religion, or socioeconomic status, we were all (ideally) conceived through pleasure, and that pleasure should accompany us throughout our entire lives.

I now invite you to celebrate your sexuality by embarking on a lifelong journey into the realm of enhanced pleasure.

May *The Boudoir Bible* accompany you and yours, every ecstatic step of the way!

BETONY VERNON
March 2019

PLATES

———o———

INTRODUCTION

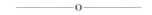

IN THE REALM
OF SEXUAL PLEASURE—
THE PATH IS THE DESTINATION

*I know that what you call "God" really exists, but not in the form you
think; God is primal cosmic energy, the love in your body, your integrity,
and your perception of the nature in you and outside of you.*

— Wilhelm Reich, "Listen, Little Man!"

I AM FREQUENTLY ASKED by curious new acquaintances how I found
myself working in the realm of sexual pleasure. It's a good question,
but one that is also guaranteed to monopolize a conversation. I
have learned to swerve around the inevitable at dinners and parties
by stating things such as "It's too long a story to go into now,"
then quickly changing the topic. But here I feel that it is not only
appropriate but also essential to reveal a few landmarks of my journey into the sexual realm. My sexual journey commenced, just
like yours did, during the innocence of my childhood—discovering
my body, enjoying sensations, playing doctor, my first kiss—and
it led, over the years that followed, to discovering new facets of
myself and my sexual identity within relationships, to the fine arts
and design world, and to the wide-open, still largely unexplored

field of sexology.

I was born in 1968 in Tazewell, Virginia, a four-square-mile patch of civilization on the Appalachian Trail nestled among thick forests, rolling farmlands, and coal-rich mountaintops. Inhabited at the time by fewer than 250 coal miners, loggers, and farmers, it was the kind of place where people went to bed and rose with the sun and where everyone knew one another—and everything about one another, too.

Two years before, my father, a helicopter pilot specializing in seeding strip mines, had decided to buy the big wooden Victorian house that would become the bastion of my childhood. Once my parents had restored and settled into their new home with what were then two daughters, my father took to the skies, and he stayed up there until it was too cold to either fly or seed. My mother essentially bore the responsibility of bringing us up on her own, but in my father's long absences, the foundations of their relationship cracked and crumbled, and by 1972 my parents were divorced.

A conservative Virginia judge granted my father full custody, a decision that was a quasi-miracle for the time and influenced by my mother's history as a civil rights activist. In February of 1960, she had been temporarily expelled from college and risked being deported back to her native Great Britain for supporting the Greensboro Four, four African-American men whose demand for equal rights at the famous sit-in at the "Whites Only" lunch counter at the Woolworth store in downtown Greensboro, North Carolina, defied racial segregation. The sit-in signaled the beginning of America's civil rights revolution, and ten years later it sparked a revolution in the Vernon family, too.

The day my mother had to leave home, I was four years old, and my sisters were two, six, and eleven. During the frigid winter months, my father raised us, but, as soon as the snow and ice started to melt and return to the rivers in the valleys, he took to the skies again. My eldest sister and a hired nanny, for a time, became our surrogate parents, but we essentially ended up raising one another. In retrospect, I am certain that this lack of parental guidance and prohibition made a deep impact on the formation of my sexual persona.

My first recollection of deriving pleasure from genital stimulation dates back to when I was very young. The inanimate object of my innocent delight dwelt in my father's study—a footstool in the shape of a miniature bull. I was told time and again that, as cute as the stool was, it was not a toy. I was allowed to sit on it, but I mustn't ride it. So only when I was certain that I would not be caught and reprimanded would I dare express the real extent of my appreciation for that leather bull, by mounting it and rocking away to my heart and body's content!

Unlike most little girls, I did not have dolls. My father was convinced that they served little more than to train girls to be mothers. (He might be right, as only one of his four daughters chose to have children.) While I did not have dolls of my own, I had a playmate who possessed a throng of Barbies, as well as Barbie's friend Skipper, her boyfriend, Ken, and an infantry of minuscule plastic babies. We spent hours in her bedroom after school, dressing and undressing Barbie and her friends. We inevitably discovered that the most exciting thing to do with Barbie and Ken was to make them have sex (and of course, make babies!). Just as it is for any healthy kid, from a very early age, emulation of adult activities was an integrated part of my playtime.

Body exploration and seeking new and different sensations of all sorts are part of everyone's childhood. I must have been about six when I finally discovered just how very different boys and girls are. A long low table in the sunroom served as the theater for our doctor-patient games. The examination consisted of first taking a look at the patient's eyes and ears, and then, with a big *ahhhhh*, the tonsils were examined. We moved down our playmate's body and listened to his or her heartbeat. Finally it was time to get a good, long look at the more intimate bits. Once "the doctor" had poked and prodded his or her "patient" to their mutual satisfaction, the roles would be reversed.

S . . . S-A . . . S-E . . . S-E-X!

A *Playboy* magazine nicked from the driver of my father's helicopter's fuel truck satisfied my growing curiosity at first, but soon I decided to go to the local library and research my newfound topic of enthrallment by looking up the subject of sex. (I'm quite sure that most of you living in the age before the Internet did the same thing.) My heart started to race as soon as I touched the brass handle on the *S* file. I pulled the long wooden drawer out, ever so slowly, and quickly shuffled through the cards . . . *S* . . . *S-A* . . . *S-E* . . . *S-E-X*! I slipped down the *S* aisle, scanning the bindings of the books until my eye caught the code and title that matched my search: *The Joy of Sex*, by Alex Comfort.

I sought out an empty study room and settled into a beanbag chair in a corner opposite the librarian's glass observation window. I turned every page of the volume as fast as I could until I found the illustrations. From time to time, I would tear my gawking eyes away from the images and make sure that the librarian was not anywhere near her window. By the time I turned the last page, I was possessed by an uncontrollable desire to take the book home, so I pressed *The Joy of Sex* against my chest and zipped my red vinyl slicker over it.

I took a deep breath and marched straight past the librarian and through the double doors. As soon as my feet hit the sidewalk, I started to run. When I finally burst through the back door of my house, I dashed straight up to my bedroom, but I didn't stuff the erotic booty under my mattress next to my *Playboy* magazine and a copy of Judy Blume's *Are You There God? It's Me, Margaret* that one of my classmates had lent to me. Instead I plopped myself down on the bed with only one thing on my mind: *The Joy of Sex*!

A FORMAL SEX EDUCATION

Though my secret library fueled my imagination, at the age of thirteen I finally received some formal sex education—or, rather, abstinence education. Like other eighth graders of that era, my classmates and I learned the basic functions of the male and female sexual apparatuses. We also learned about sexually transmitted diseases in gory detail, along with the biology of the menstrual cycle, ovulation, and spermatozoa—all information related to making babies. The pleasures and benefits of a healthy sex life were never mentioned. But thanks to my secret collection of erotica and the uncensored reports of my older sisters' experiences, I had no doubt there was a lot more to sex than dangerous diseases and making babies.

During my first year in high school, I secretly dated a senior. Every time this young man took my hand, even just to accompany me down the hall to a class, I got hot flashes and butterflies in my stomach. We engaged in a great deal of heavy petting and panting in his car or in my favorite spot, a field on the other side of the forest. One evening, I came home just late enough to make my father's imagination run wild. In reality I had not been up to any girl-boy mischief. I had simply lost track of time while studying with a friend. While looking me straight in the eyes, he warned, "Beware, my child. If you play, you are likely to pay!" This cryptic warning, alongside the swelling bellies of two of my classmates, served to inspire a sense of self-preservation, but I would never forget my father's use of the word "play." For the next two years, I remained an adventurous and playful virgin.

On my sixteenth birthday, following the advice of my eldest sister, I gave myself a gift: my first Planned Parenthood appointment. The gynecologist asked me if I was sexually active. I told her that though I had not gone "all the way," there was someone that I liked enough to do so with, and that was why I was there. She examined me, then gave me a prescription for the birth-control pill. Freed by modern science, I was liberated from the chains of chastity exactly one month later by that chosen man. A few years older than I was, he had no idea that I gave him my virginity, or how happy I was to get "it" over and done with!

One day he introduced me to a friend of his who owned a vintage clothing shop. About three minutes later I had a part-time job, if you could call it that. Street Theatre was more than just a shop—it was a 1980s destination. Musicians, bikers, post-punk rockers, fetishists, and fashionistas came from up and down America's East Coast to buy the coolest, sexiest, darkest, most daring looks we could possibly concoct. Street Theatre also carried a large selection of English leather: fuck-me pumps, metal-studded bras and belts, buckled boots, handcuffs, masks, chaps, erotic straitjackets and body harnesses, and other accoutrements of the closely aligned worlds of alternative fashion and BDSM (the matrix of bondage and discipline, sadism and masochism).

When the shop was empty, we watched Swedish pornographic videos in the back room while mending new entries from the secondhand stores that we plundered on a regular basis. Part of my job was to work a look that was representative of the shop's aesthetics. I was happy to wear anything that confined and defined my *Faster, Pussycat! Kill! Kill!* curves. I loved the constrictive powers of Victorian corsets and black lace girdles and 1940s and 1950s lingerie, and seamed stockings and torpedo bras became the essence of my wardrobe when I was not attending school. In retrospect, I realize that I had stumbled upon a different kind of loving thanks to my interest in fashion.

There was one browser who came into the shop nearly every day. There was something dangerously sexy about his tattoos, his devilish beard, and the scent of his leather riding gear. The passes he made at me over the jewelry counter flustered me, as did the rumble of his low-riding bike pulling into the parking lot next to the shop. He was mature, pushing forty, and I was going on eighteen the day I accepted his offer to take a ride.

Sitting behind him on his motorcycle was empowering. I had never, in my short life, ever felt more grown-up, womanly, or free. But as he pulled into the driveway of his beachfront apartment, I felt my heart skip a beat, and by the time I was standing in his living room, it was racing so fast and hard that I thought I might faint. He offered me a beer, put on some music, and we perched on the railing of his balcony, which looked out over the thunderous waves of the Atlantic. We chatted just long enough for me to pull myself together, and then he kissed me, putting his hand on my thigh, and we abandoned the balcony for his bedroom.

We were writhing in a frenzy of kisses and caresses when he abruptly pulled away and looked into my eyes. Then he slowly pushed my wrists up over my head, held them down, and whispered in my ear, "You are a naughty girl, aren't you? I think you need a spanking!" Laughing hysterically, I tried to escape, but he grabbed me, rolled me playfully over his knees, and proceeded to give me exactly what he thought I deserved.

At first I resisted and tried again to escape, but after a few perfectly targeted strokes, I realized that his goal was not to hurt me— but to please me. My decision to let go and comply with this new game was anything but conscious; my body changed my mind because I was thoroughly enjoying myself! I was happy to let him alternate between spanking my now-rosy cheeks and rubbing my crotch. When he finally allowed me to roll over, I attempted to express my appreciation, but he made it very clear that my pleasure was his.

Then, without taking his hands off my body, he asked me if I had ever been restrained. Without the slightest hesitation, I lied, "Yes, of course!" And before Little Miss Know-It-All could think about what she was allowing to happen, her wrists were buckled into a pair of leather cuffs, and she was bound, spread-eagled against the bedroom door, her cheek against its cool wood.

Thanks to those back-room porn breaks at the shop, I had a vague idea of what could happen, and I had good reason to be nervous, since the only bondage scenes I was familiar with involved moaning masochists and seriously relentless sadists.

But I was lucky. This man was well intentioned and skilled, not only with his hands but also with the soft leather flogger he took up for our pleasure. He never once overstepped my limits, and he checked in with me constantly to make sure I was okay. I felt safe and gradually handed over the reins of my pleasure. It wasn't long before I understood that he was enjoying my initiation just as much as I was. That was the summer of 1986, a few weeks before I left Norfolk to study fine arts at Virginia Commonwealth University in Richmond, Virginia.

I took the liberal arts program at the university as seriously as I took my sexual liberty, in spite of the glaring reality of HIV. My young generation was the last to feel free enough to engage in orgiastic debauchery and promiscuous sex without using barriers. Fortunately, I made it through, unscathed, what I now recognize to have been a dangerously carefree period of sexual exploration. When I think back on those years of polyamorous generosity, I count my blessings.

A FABULOUSLY GENEROUS LOVER

During my sophomore year, I met another man who would make a very important impression on my sexual perspective. The first time I succumbed to his call for courtship was also the first time I experienced a sexual high. A fabulously generous lover, he insisted on proving we could both be multiorgasmic. By the time I had climaxed for the third time, I believed him. It was a long night of lovemaking; our bodies fused, and we left all earthly things behind.

The next morning, we shared a hot bath and got dressed. After serving me a bacchanalian fruit plate, he gave me a private reading of some of his favorite poems, and then—with a glint in his eye—he commanded, "Now take off everything but your shoes, and sit on that chair!" His tone was playfully stern, and so I happily obeyed. Taking off his clothes, he stretched out on the bed in the exact position where I had spent a good part of the evening and announced, "I am in the mood to switch. It's your turn to take care of me." I went over to the bed, nervously proceeded to buckle his hands and feet into the soft leather cuffs that were attached to the bedposts, and we resumed our journey. I did not exit the gates of Paradise until twenty-four hours later, and if I had not had a French class that Monday morning, I would have stayed exactly where I was.

As I walked across the campus, I felt elated, as if I had done drugs. It took me the entire day to get my head together, and when I finally did come down from my sexual high, I realized I was hooked on the effects of multiple orgasms, extended playtime, restraint, and full-body stimulation. It was through this special union that I came to understand the relevance of initiation, as well as the importance of being a proactive lover. The extent of my capacity for pleasure had been revealed. This relationship, which endured about a year, made a distinct and lasting impact on my sexual development.

In 1990, a few days after I received a bachelor's degree in art history with a minor in metalsmithing from Virginia Commonwealth University, I said my last good-byes to the couple I was dating at the time, and I boarded a plane for Italy. I was twenty-one years old, I had a one-way ticket in hand, and my destination was Florence, where a position teaching goldsmithing awaited me. I had packed one very large suitcase and a carry-on toolbox full of files, pliers of various shapes and sizes, a saw, sharp shears, and a few other necessities of jewelry making. While I was already fairly aware of what my sexual needs and desires were, I hadn't even the faintest idea where my love for the arts and jewelry was going to lead me.

I started teaching at Art Studio Fuji to college students studying abroad from around the world. I learned Italian and pursued the refinement of my craft by apprenticing to various Florentine masters of age-old techniques like *repoussé*, inlay, enameling, stonecutting, and stone setting. In 1992, I launched my first handmade jewelry line at Luisa Via Roma, a renowned high-end fashion retailer in Florence. A limited number of boutiques from the United States and Japan followed. The collection included a family of objects that I playfully called "Sado-Chic." Inspired by *The Story of O*, this collection would spark a series of life-changing events.

In 1995, I moved from Florence to Milan to obtain my master's degree in industrial design at Domus Academy. I also reopened my atelier in a loft on the outskirts of the city, where I continued to develop my jewelry collections for fashion retailers as well as a series of "one-offs" for my own very personal pleasure. I called these useful objects my "jewel-tools." They were a luxurious response to the implements of the sex-toy industry, which satisfied neither my lust for quality materials nor my sense of aesthetics. I never dared to show the gold and silver jewel-tools to the accessory buyers who came to my studio. I was fully aware that I was ahead of my time in terms of retail; any item with an obviously sexual function would be considered anything *but* chic by the fashion world. At the time, fashion could be sexy but not explicitly related to sex.

By the end of 2000, the Boudoir Box, the deluxe leather travel case that I designed to transport my erotic collections, was complete. I made my first trip with the Boudoir Box to New York City, then to London via Paris. While potential retail venues were still out of sight, the ability of the Boudoir Box to turn any hotel room into a seductive showroom was proven effective. The group of private collectors for my erotic designs grew, essentially like-minded friends and friends of friends who were as interested as I was in the art of loving.

After the Twin Towers in Manhattan were attacked on September 11, 2001, I finally found the courage to come out of creative hiding and follow my vision. If I were to continue to design anything at all, it would be openly and in the name of love and sexual pleasure. A few weeks after the disaster, I naively presented the Paradise Found Fine Erotic Jewelry collection to my regular retail clients during Fashion Week in Paris. I can still hear myself trying to explain the concept of the collection to the accessory buyers of institutions like Barneys of New York City, Liberty of London, and Kashiyama Tokyo, as well as other independent boutiques that had carried my jewelry lines.

On the first day of sales, I earnestly attempted to enlighten these commercial entities with a redefinition of the function of jewelry. Might we not discreetly enrich its ornamental purpose with the power to please all the senses—and not just the sense of sight? I expounded on the value of sexual satisfaction and the benefits of providing sensations that engage the entire body, genitals included. I told them that the collection was an invitation to my collectors to explore new ways to make love, emphasizing my desire to bring a novel sense of aesthetics to the sexual experience through the use of noble metals.

Some of them told me, with disconcerted expressions, that I was brave; some, however affectionately, let me know that they thought I was crazy. Others wrinkled up their noses with a hint of disgust, regretfully expressing the hope that my next season would be different, because as much as they found the collection "interesting," they could not sell objects "of this nature" in their shops. One client whispered in my ear that she was surprised that I was so "kinky."

As the days passed without any sales, I tried editing my sales pitch. I used terms such as "empowerment," "holistic," and "awareness" in an attempt to get my point across and to avoid having my creative initiatives pigeonholed as S&M. I placed particular emphasis on the fact that most of the jewel-tools could be worn discreetly as jewelry for any occasion, because their function to provide pleasure was disguised within their sleek silver and gold forms. But by the end of the week, I managed to place only one order with my favorite client in Japan.

I had naively presumed that my retailers, widely considered to be on the cutting edge of fashion, would grasp my concept and embrace the collection. But it turned out that I was terribly wrong. The outcome of the week was a disconcerting realization that not everyone viewed—at least not openly—the sexual experience as I did.

It was thanks to this utter failure that I realized I had some very serious work to do, and I understood it could not be done at my drawing table or jeweler's bench alone. If I wanted to render my Paradise Found Fine Erotic Jewelry collection accessible to a wider public, this would require that I integrate the foundations of my sexual knowledge and experience into the totality of my life and assume the role of educator in order to expand people's limited viewpoints on sex.

I began to examine sexual perspectives and identities in all cultures. I studied psychology and explored sexual history in the hopes of better understanding why humans categorize and pigeonhole themselves and one another. I delved into my own sexual etiology (something I encourage you to do as well) in an attempt to discover how the sexual experiences of my childhood and my adolescence had shaped my sex life as an adult. Then, departing from my personal experiences, I accumulated research material while consulting for the individuals and couples who collected my jewel-tools, which in turn came to represent the bridge to my mission to enhance humanity's sexual understanding and thereby well-being, just as my vision had promised.

I developed a series of classes, and in November 2002 I initiated my first group salon, "Bettering Your Sexual Skills," in London. My host was Samantha Roddick, the founder of the world's first female-friendly, luxury erotic boutique, Coco de Mer, and the first retailer of my Paradise Found Fine Erotic Jewelry collection. Her approach to sex was holistic. She understood the relevance of honoring our sexuality with materials that are as body safe as they are beautifully crafted, as poetic as they are functional. We hit it off instantly.

Thirty participants had settled into the leather-covered conference room of Soho House by the time I took my place on the stage. I had butterflies in my stomach because, up until then, I had only initiated private collectors, on a one-on-one basis, into the techniques and tools of what I called "The Paradise Found Sexual Ceremony."

My eyes scanned the room. I had been informed that the group was composed of lovers from all walks of life, including a journalist, who, perching on the edge of her seat in the middle of the front row, steadied a bright red notepad on her knees. With a pang of disappointment, I realized that there was only one man in the group, although I had not limited attendance to women, as I believe that women and men—of all sexual orientations—must progress together toward sexual enlightenment. This lone, nervous man had chosen a chair in the farthest corner of the room. When our eyes met, he sank down lower into its soft leather embrace. I tried to comfort him with a smile but only provoked a flush of embarrassment that did not fade until I began to speak:

"Welcome, and thank you all for coming today," I began. "I have to admit that I am moved. I consider this occasion as much a privilege as it is an exciting sign that our sexual horizons are expanding again . . ."

PARADISE FOUND

Only fifty years ago, attendees of my Sexual Skills salons would have been putting their private and professional lives at risk. Things have changed since the 1950s; I have much to thank for this, including the revolutionary research of many brave people, such as the American scientist Dr. Alfred Kinsey.

Dr. Kinsey's mission was to demonstrate and thus convince people that sex was good, natural, and wholesome, and that sexual satisfaction was essential to their happiness. By disseminating sexual knowledge and understanding, he publicly contradicted the Judeo-Christian association of sexual pleasure with the transgression of divine law and damnation. Without being fully aware of it, Dr. Kinsey dropped a sociocultural "sex bomb," and his commitment to his cause contributed to the sexual liberation movement of the 1960s. His stalwart convictions led him to be repeatedly arrested, the persecution bringing him to nervous exhaustion, but by 1970, many sexual taboos had been kicked aside.

In 1971, America's president Richard Nixon had repealed the most sexually repressive elements of the Comstock laws, state and federal restrictions on what was deemed "obscene," and the liberation movement began to flourish legally. Revolutionary figures such as Dr. William Masters and Virginia Johnson, Betty Dodson, Annie Sprinkle, Shere Hite, and Alex Comfort openly explored sexual frontiers that had hitherto been denied access by the establishment, and countless sex workers, researchers, doctors, psychologists, therapists, artists, and women and men of all sexual orientations joined the movement.

Abstinence and repression were traded for pleasure, and the infernal repercussions of carnal sin (according to Judeo-Christian credo) turned to ash in the flames of passion. Nurtured by the widespread acceptance of birth control, the decade to follow would mark the most sexually liberated era in history since the height of the ancient Greek and Roman civilizations.

But although the enlightened Dr. Kinsey and his successors managed to stretch the parameters of what Westerners once considered acceptable sexual behavior, even today many people continue to limit the definition of "normal" sex to predominantly genitally orientated forms of stimulation, which are initiated merely to enable penetration and provoke the release of sexual tension through orgasm. Extra-genital stimulation, on the other hand, is still commonly judged to be abnormal, or categorized as S&M, in spite of the fact that the implements of full-body stimulation, like those who appreciate them, are no longer confined to the underground.

What I seek to dismantle in my Sexual Skills salons are the die-hard taboos associated with the categorizations of "normal" sexual behavior and with the related derivation of pleasure through extra-genital stimulation. Founded on restrictive Judeo-Christian morals, the codes of "normal"—and thus acceptable—sexual conduct were consolidated into medical terms at the turn of the nineteenth century by the German neuropsychiatrist Dr. Richard von Krafft-Ebing. In his still-famous and highly influential work *Psychopathia Sexualis,* published in 1886, more than two hundred variations of non-procreative sexual behavior are painstakingly described and essentially denounced as deviant. Some of the Victorian ideals that Krafft-Ebing propagated still sound familiar to many of us: "proper" and therefore "normal" women are passive; any act that results in pleasure for pleasure's sake is sexually deviant, including masturbation, anal sex, same-sex encounters, and eroticized extra-genital stimulation; and sexual deviance is a disease that can, and should, be cured.

By the mid-1900s, the same treatments that were prescribed to "cure" criminals and the mentally ill were being prescribed to cure the "disease" of sexual deviance—treatments including lobotomies, electroshock therapy, and clitoridectomies. Krafft-Ebing's *Psychopathia Sexualis* served as the foundation for sexual research up until the 1950s, and by criminalizing the principle of sexual pleasure, it helped to codify the condemning behavioral restrictions that shaped—and continue to influence—the Western world's sexual perceptions today.

In order to shed the remnants of these oppressive codes of conduct, we must first delineate new parameters of normalcy. According to the philosophy of Paradise Found, any form or degree of erotic stimulation (genital or extra-genital) that is performed between consenting adults (whatever their gender or sexual orientation) and that does not infringe upon anyone's desires, rights, wishes, or innocence is to be considered natural and acceptable sexual behavior.

This philosophy is key to the Paradise Found Sexual Ceremony. By creating a ritualized context for sexual exploration, extending the duration of the time of the sexual encounter, and engaging the entire body as a sexual whole, the ceremony aims to broaden the horizons of pleasure beyond that which may be experienced through "normal," everyday sex. And a note on the word "normal": to avoid the discriminatory undertones that the word implies, I coined the term "predominantly genitally oriented" (PGO) sex and will use it throughout *The Boudoir Bible*. (After all, no one fits the cookie-cutter category of "normal" . . . once you really get to know him or her.)

PGO sex typically results in fleeting encounters that last from three to fifteen minutes—we may from this conclude that overemphasis upon the genitals, and in particular the male genitals, is the number-one cause of "fast sex." While fast sex may provide for the superficial release of sexual tension (and there are times in life that permit little more), such fleeting, genitals-localized pleasures, as a steady regime, do nothing to reveal anyone's true pleasure potential. More often than not, fast sex has the tendency to reduce the sacred union to a compulsive, mechanical act that leaves one or both partners in an emotional void, physically insatiate, or utterly frustrated. Beyond a procreative function, this kind of sexual interaction serves a very limited purpose.

The Paradise Found Sexual Ceremony presents the antithesis to PGO sex. In order to reap the benefits it can provide, lovers will be obliged to put phallocentric role models and their allied behavioral patterns aside, as these do nothing to cultivate the full extent of our pleasure capacity, nor do they permit a sexual ritual to evolve. It is through the simple act of bettering sexual skills that lovers will learn to elaborate rituals that may unfold over hours, if not days. The longer the ritual lasts, the greater its overall effects are likely to be. The ecstatic results induce a sense of psychophysiological well-being that continue to radiate long after the ceremony's end.

THE PLEASURE PALETTE

Self-knowledge is key to developing one's potential in sex as well as in life, and so *The Boudoir Bible* enters "The Gardens of Earthly Delight" with the chapter "The Anatomy of Desire: A Comparative Approach," which is an enlightening map to your own—and your partner's—body geography. You will find that the similarities between the male and female genitals are as marked as their differences.

During the Paradise Found Sexual Ceremony, penetration does not serve as the means to an end but as a pleasure practiced over and over again, throughout the ceremony's duration. Similarly, orgasm is not the only reason to initiate the ritual (though it is one of its greatest rewards, as described in the chapter "Enhancing the Orgasm: Coaxing the Sexual Vibration."). The entire body, not just the genitals, is engaged as a sexual, sensual whole.

By removing the sole focus of attention from the genitals, and alternating between genital and extra-genital, or full-body, stimulation, you can experience and provide a wider range of ecstatic sensations. This radically extends the duration of the sexual ceremony and enhances your overall perception of pleasure therein. By inviting sexual tension to mount gradually over an extended period of arousal, your body, mind, and spirit will become charged with the sexual vibration. Regardless of gender or sexual orientation, extended "playtime" is the heartbeat of the Sexual Ceremony.

The ability of men to delay the ejaculation reflex during orgasm is crucial to the progression of the ceremony. The chapter "Riding the Orgasmic Wave: Male Ejaculation Control" explores many techniques that both facilitate the delay of the ejaculation reflex and build sexual tension. The chapter "Navigating the Sacred River: Female Emissions," unveils the Holy Grail of female orgasmic potential, the G-spot. Techniques of genital and anal stimulation are described throughout this first section of *The Boudoir Bible*, including a special dedication to the much-maligned "rosebud" in "The Anthems of Anal Sex: From Hygiene to Heavenly Pleasures." These techniques will lead lovers to unprecedented heights of pleasure during the Paradise Found Sexual Ceremony.

Once the true extent of the body's pleasure capacity is unveiled, PGO "quickies" will no longer be a sexual mainstay. As the saying goes, "Variety is the spice of life," and our sex lives are no exception. The more varied our pleasure palette becomes, the more options and possibilities we have to choose from, and the more creative, less compulsive, and deeply satisfying our sexual relations will be.

SACRED SEX

Central to the philosophy of Paradise Found is the concept and practice of sacred sex. In some people's minds, the association of the terms "ceremony" and "sacred" with the subject of sex might conjure up hedonistic, "anything goes" visions of salacious lechery. But the Paradise Found Sexual Ceremony—as any sexual activity, for that matter—has a very firm limit: it should *never* infringe upon the wishes, desires, rights, or innocence of anyone involved. Ceremonies are organized to honor special moments, people, and events, and the Paradise Found Sexual Ceremony is no exception.

Ceremonies take place at predetermined times and places, and like any other art form, they incorporate tools and techniques that amplify the final result and the overall impact of the ritualized expression. As master voice coach Patsy Rodenburg, who uses the works of Shakespeare as her pedagogical medium, explains in her book *The Second Circle: How to Use Positive Energy for Success in Every Situation*: "Rituals prepare your body for the sacred, and they release your energy, feelings, and thoughts. They open the body to receive wisdom and clarity, and to release and purge negativity."

No matter the genre or the motivation, ceremonies mark the difference between the ordinary and the extraordinary, between the sacred and the profane, and the concept of sexual ritual is by all no means new. Pre-Judeo-Christian cultures integrated the sacred sexual union and religion through fertility cults, as means to both venerate the gods and procure transcendental pleasures. The sexual ritual was used to push the limits of existence, to crack the doors to mysterious realms that lie beyond the earthly confines of the human body. Body and spirit were not considered to be opposing forces in conflict until the advent of monotheism.

Beyond the borders of Western culture, the philosophical disciplines of Taoism in China (circa 600 B.C.) and Tantric Buddhism in India (circa 300 B.C.) evolved highly sophisticated rituals of erotic loving. Deeply influenced by the fertility cults that preceded them, both the Taoists and the Tantrists viewed the sexual union in the context of a spiritual aspiration. The ultimate goal of their ecstatic rituals was neither to release sexual tension nor to merely procreate, but to achieve oneness—with one's partner, one's self, and with the entire universe. Sexual satisfaction was associated with overall well-being and longevity. Sex was venerated for its capacity to heighten one's perceptions and to potentially lead to the attainment of spiritual enlightenment.

The Taoists used the sexual vibration to establish and maintain the balance between the masculine and feminine forces. One of the principal goals of their intimate endeavors was to open and align the energy centers of the body through euphoric pleasure. The Tantrists also used the healing flux of the sexual vibration. To disintegrate energy blocks that negatively affect body, mind, and spirit, they sought to align the body's energy centers, the *chakras*, or "wheels" of vital energy, as they are called in Sanskrit. Both disciplines developed techniques to facilitate ejaculation control in order to prolong the duration of the sexual union and thereby channel the sexual vibration to ecstatic effect, both in and beyond the boudoir. Lack of sexual skill was considered detrimental to both the satisfaction and the overall well-being of the sexually mature aspirant.

In the West, the ancient Greeks also developed highly evolved sexual ceremonies; their ritual endeavors were similar to those of the Tantrists and Taoists, in that the ultimate goal was illumination. They used various tools and techniques in order to provoke frenzy, which ideally would induce what they termed *ektasis*. *Ektasis* was appreciated as a path toward sexual satisfaction and for its inducement of the loss of ego. This state would eventually lead to *enthousiasmos*, or the possession of a mere mortal by a god. The

Greeks believed that this divine encounter, or *Logos*, was the embodied creative principle that sets all life into motion, as well as the culmination of the sexual experience. Like the practitioners of the Eastern disciplines of erotic loving, the Greeks ritualized their sexual endeavors as a means to guarantee the prosperity of the individual, the spiritual evolution of the people, and the welfare of the community as a whole.

LOVE DRUGS

There is a scientific explanation for our ancient ancestors' association of sex with universal oneness, divine encounters, and transcendence: the effects of pleasure-enhancing hormones and endorphins. Mutual attraction strums the pleasure centers of the brain, which respond by transmitting signals to various parts of the body, including the endocrine system. The endocrine system is composed of eight major glands—the pituitary (which works in tandem with the hypothalamus), the pineal, the thyroid (with its accompanying parathyroid), the thymus, the adrenal glands, the pancreas, and the gonads, or the testes in men and the ovaries in women. When we are sexually aroused, the function of the endocrine glands is turned up a notch or two, and the production and release into the bloodstream of hormones and pleasure-enhancing endorphins are increased. The locations of the endocrine glands correspond to the locations of the seven principal chakras, according to Ayurveda, the traditional Hindu system of medicine.

The pituitary gland lies deep inside the seat of the brain, and its corresponding chakra, the "third eye," is located between the eyes. The pituitary gland regulates the secretion of several hormones, including oxytocin, a.k.a. the "love hormone." This natural antidepressant is associated with intimate bonding, so it is not surprising that an orgasm causes the flow of this hormone to surge. Two people who are genuinely sexually attracted to each other produce more pleasure-enhancing hormones than people who are not, and this is one of the many reasons why being in love can feel so good.

The pituitary gland also produces endorphins. The term "endorphin" is a combination of "endogenous" (meaning "originating from the body") and "morphine." Endorphins have a chemical structure that resembles that of opiates, and just like any other mind-altering substance, the body's natural "love drugs" can alter the perception of body, time, and space as well as increase tolerance to pain and incite feelings of pleasure and euphoria. Endorphins also provoke that uncontrollable sense of dependency, if not downright addiction, that is intrinsic to new love.

The pituitary gland works in synchronicity with a neighboring organ called the hypothalamus. The hypothalamus not only secretes hormones and synthesizes endorphins but also serves as a link, via the pituitary gland, to both the nervous system and the endocrine system. The hypothalamus produces the hormone dopamine, which is known to open doors to new sensory dimensions by inducing a "drifty" sense of happiness and serenity.

Some of the hormones that are produced readily during sexual arousal work as neurotransmitters—they "stroke" the pleasure centers of the brain. For example, the neurotransmitter norepinephrine, a natural amphetamine, induces sensations of euphoria and enhances our overall perception of pleasure, including that of the orgasm. Norepinephrine is produced in the adrenal glands, which are positioned atop the kidneys. The root chakra, located in the perineum between the genitals and the anus, corresponds with both the adrenal glands and the gonads. The adrenal glands also produce adrenaline, which triggers the well-known "fight or flight" response.

"Fast" PGO sexual encounters cannot incite endorphin/hormone elation, while the skilled elaboration of the Paradise Found Sexual Ceremony *will* prompt endocrine synchronicity. Over extended and intense periods of lovemaking, the inebriating effects of the body's "love drugs" become increasingly evident. Rituals that involve a combination of genital and extra-genital stimulation are capable of inducing trancelike states that have been described as an out-of-body experience, a high, or "sexual flight."

The chemistry of pleasure is a fascinating topic that deserves more space than can be afforded here. But it is important to mention that unlike chemical or artificial mind-altering substances, the body's natural love drugs are known to revive body, mind, and spirit. They cannot produce negative side effects, as long as lovers avoid getting so high that they unintentionally break limits that have been established before the ritual begin.

THE SPARK OF DESIRE

Just as the brain increases endocrine activity during arousal, it also emits varying electrical frequencies. Understanding the activity of alpha and theta brain waves in relation to pleasure helps to further explain why our forefathers and foremothers considered sex to be sacred.

The alpha brain-wave frequency is emitted in association with the creative forces of passion, intuition, inspiration, emotions, day-dreams, fantasy, and desire, nurturing every single creative impulse into being, including the enigmatic, seemingly uncontrollable libido itself. When your sexual desire is sparked by the senses, by a fantasy, or simply by the way someone looks at you, the most primal recesses of the right side of the brain perceive an impulse and activate the emission of the alpha brain-wave frequency. The same frequency is also emitted during the stage of rapid eye movement, or REM, sleep, when alpha waves are also present. During sexual arousal, the dance of the alpha frequency is radically amplified in both the receiver and the provider of sensations, and even more so if sensations are being administered in a ritualized context. The alpha brain-wave frequency is associated with calm, focused, trancelike states.

Then, as sexual pleasure peaks, the brain-wave frequency switches to theta, which induces a brief but ultra-deep cerebral slumber, even as the body is writhing under the uncontrollable influence of the orgasmic wave. The theta frequency is not only emitted during orgasm, but also during sleep when little or no dream activity occurs, as well as when one is under hypnosis or in a trance.

Practitioners of meditation learn to trigger the theta brain-wave frequency through the mastery of the mind. Practitioners of yoga attain similar results via positions, known as *asana,* coupled with breath-control techniques, or *pranayama.* Skilled lovers will incur similar benefits, and have all the more fun doing so, by charging each other's bodies, minds, and spirits with the sexual vibration over extended periods of ritualized playtime.

The combined effects of orgasm, increased endorphin/hormone production, and the emission of the alpha and theta brain-wave frequencies permit me to describe the Paradise Found Sexual Ceremony as an erotic meditation. It is in this spirit that the chapters "The Pleasure Priority: Timing the Ritual" and "Eros and Order: Erecting the Temple" invite you to prioritize the role that sexual pleasure plays in your physical, emotional, and spiritual well-being. The chapter "Ascent to Paradise: Orchestrating the Senses" describes how to fine-tune the senses in order to heighten their pleasure-providing function. The chapter "The Joy of Play: The Roles of Provider and Receiver" encourages you to go beyond the limits of categories and to communicate and take responsibility for your deepest wishes and desires. These chapters in "Paradise Found: The Sexual Ceremony" will help you acquire the sexual understanding that permits you to develop and refine your skills, and thus begin to experience heightened degrees of sexual satisfaction. Like the disciplines of yoga and meditation, the Paradise Found Sexual Ceremony is a catalyst for our overall health and happiness.

The ideas outlined thus far in these pages were actually the introductory contents of my first Paradise Found Sexual Skills Salon in London. What followed at that salon was the opening of the Boudoir Box. The chapters in "Transcendental Techniques," from "Expanding the Sexual Arena: Implements of Ecstasy" to "X Marks the Sweet Spot: Erotic Flagellation," correspond to my demonstration of the implements of desire and techniques of full-body stimulation, as well as the dos and don'ts of these tools and techniques. Both the salon and *The Boudoir Bible* conclude with "Back to Reality: Coming Down," which emphasizes the relevance of reveling in the afterglow together while allowing the endorphin high to subside. My goal with every salon—and with *The Boudoir Bible*—is to inspire with the possibility of enriching one's sex life and relationships.

What I learned from the first experience of sharing the philosophy of my Paradise Found Sexual Ceremony with a group of open-minded individuals continues to motivate and influence my work today. At the end of that very first salon in London, the journalist who had scribbled the whole time in her red notebook asked me if she could publish an article about her experience that day. I consented, and she thanked me with a hug, exclaiming, "We really should have learned about all of this at school!" She was one of many people who inspired me to write the book you are now holding in your hands.

———o———

The

GARDENS OF EARTHLY DELIGHT

**In which sexual self-knowledge becomes
the key to the arts of ecstatic love and ascending
to the gates of Paradise.**

IF WE LEAVE our sexual gratification to the chance determinants of
love or instinct, we will discover that neither guarantees our
evolution toward becoming fully realized sexual beings. Many people
still believe the age-old myths that intense sexual pleasure is the
natural result of true love and that learning more about pleasure,
beyond the lessons of experience itself, obliterates the ineffable
magic and mystery of the sexual union. Nothing could be further

from the truth. Do not confound a lack of sexual knowledge with magic and mystery. Realizing our sexual identity involves a lifetime's worth of exploration and discovery, and the adventure that our sex lives represent will be all the more exciting and gratifying if we are equipped with sexual knowledge and skill. Deep satisfaction is the foundation—and sexual knowledge and skill the keystones— upon which healthy sexual relations are built.

Often adults proclaim that they are not creative. If you are one of these adults, remember that in each and every child an artist dwells, and that creative child was once also you. Sex is one of the most creative experiences that you can possibly indulge in as an adult. Become the artist of your sexual destiny!

After all, true masters of any creative endeavor—be they painters, sculptors, musicians, or gourmet chefs—are recognized for their ability to stroke the subtle and refined chords of the inner spirit and, through their art, charge others' perceptions with their own heightened sense of aesthetics. Skill, when coupled with a good dose of desire and passion, marks the difference between merely bringing creative acts to fruition and creating a masterpiece.

UNITING IN THE GARDEN

Human beings unite in the garden of sexual delight for many reasons: for pure animalistic fun and pleasure, for self-expression, for adventure, and for the intensity that is the sexual experience. We also seek that sense of deep intimacy, communication, and oneness with another that sex alone can provide; we long to truly abandon ourselves to our lovers and garner the pleasure we naturally merit and that our bodies are ultimately designed to provide.

Obviously, a harmonious sexual unity depends on a combination of factors that go beyond knowledge and skill. The degree to which partners are emotionally connected radically influences the final outcome of any sexual endeavor. The more intimately we are bound together, the more we are likely to listen to and seek to satisfy each other's needs, desires, and fantasies. This being said, lovers who decide to transcend the doldrums of everyday sex through the Paradise Found Sexual Ceremony do not have to be in love. Nor do they have to be in a monogamous relationship—consolidated loving relationships that ideally permit the safe exchange of bodily fluids are simply not always on the menu. However, partners should be open to experiencing the emotional connection that deep sexual satisfaction instills, whether that connection lasts for one night or for the rest of their lives. Lovers ought to be like-minded and consent to exploring and expanding their sexual, sensory limits together in a ritualized context. Trust and respect are essential ingredients to the positive outcome: a mutually enriching sexual encounter.

Open, honest communication has a positive impact on the sexual experience. By discussing their needs, limits, and desires, lovers can swerve around the negative effects of performance pressure and avoid sexual delusions. Good communication also reduces the risk of overstepping each other's limits.

An important word on limits: they should not be considered faults or defects. Lovers think they know themselves and each other, but as our sexuality evolves, our limits also change. Limits may, rather, be viewed as potentially ecstatic and liberating "learning curves."

For many of us, communicating openly about sex may be a source of embarrassment or even great pain. Try not to judge yourself or your lover, and when you feel ready, take the initiative. You may be pleasantly surprised at just how willingly the people you care about listen and communicate. And, in fact, communicating about sex can be a bonding force. Broaching intimate or even seemingly delicate topics with your partner may open new channels of communication as well as doors to unexplored sexual domains.

Before proceeding further, it's important to broach the anything-but-hot topic of sexual health. Unless it is used in reference to solo masturbation, the expression "safe sex" is an oxymoron. A more accurate description is "safer sex." These days, the fact is that no matter how lovers fulfill their needs, the sexual union entails a certain degree of risk, be it physical or emotional. Prior to participating in any form of sexual exchange, new lovers are obliged to evaluate (and, when necessary, communicate) the potential dangers, repercussions, and material consequences of their behavior.

Sexually transmitted diseases, a.k.a. STDs, rarely make front-page news anymore, and so some people believe that they are no longer a potential threat. They are fooled by a disconcerting—and ultimately dangerous—nonchalance generated by the lack of reliable, readily available information about sexual health. The fact is that while most STDs can be cured, there is still neither a vaccine nor permanent alleviation of the fatal effects of the retrovirus HIV (human immunodeficiency virus), which causes AIDS (acquired immune-deficiency syndrome). This being said, encouraging advances are being made in regards to HIV prevention. In 2012 the U.S. Food and Drug Administration approved Truvada—the first pre-exposure prophylaxis (PrEP). For high-risk individuals who are HIV negative, this antiretroviral pharmaceutical has proven effective in HIV prevention. The pill is taken daily, much like oral contraception for women, and is best used in combination with condoms and other safe-sex practices to ensure greater protection.

At the beginning of the 1980s, HIV and AIDS signaled an abrupt deviation in humanity's sexual evolution. This disease has inflicted greater social, emotional, and physical barriers upon our sex lives than any religious or governing power has ever managed to impose. The castrating effects of HIV and AIDS may soon be halted with the diffusion of accurate sexual information and pre-exposure pro-phylaxis pharmaceuticals like Truvada. However, the use of the con-dom will also need to become as universal as its fame.

Despite medical advances in the treatment of HIV and AIDS, disease-free individuals who are not in monogamous relationships with disease-free partners must take precautions. Avoid putting even the shadow of a doubt over your own well-being or that of your part-ner(s) by using barriers such as condoms and dams when engaging in sexual activity that involves the potential exchange of bodily fluids other than saliva. While sex with barriers might not seem as psy-chologically all encompassing as sex with someone you trust and without these barriers, I cannot overemphasize the fact that the exchange of bodily fluids is a luxury reserved for monogamous, dis-ease-free partners.

In addition, condoms and dams actually have many advantages. Beyond avoiding the exchange of blood, sperm, and vaginal fluids and, therefore, the spread of STDs, they permit us to experience sexual satisfaction beyond the safety of monogamy or the solitude of masturbation. They prevent unwanted pregnancies and allow for multiple partners. Finally, they provide the psychological security that is necessary in order to abandon ourselves to the sexual realm.

A Word on Condoms

Even though barriers are the best way to practice safer sex, they must be used properly and with unfailing discipline in order to be effective against possible dangers:

- Never use the same condom twice. This rule also applies to con-doms used on dilettos or vibrators.
- Do not wear two condoms at once. This practice does *not* lead to "even more protection," but rather to the likelihood of both condoms breaking.

· Wear the correct size of condom. A condom that is too small is uncomfortable and has a very good chance of breaking. A condom that is too large is likely to slip off inside your partner. So find the right size, and stock up!

· Do not use oil-based lubricants. Oil is not latex friendly!

Know your health status, whether you are sexually active or not. If you are not perfectly well, avoid acts that would put your partner or yourself at further risk. Communicate openly—do not count on body language or on whether or not someone "looks healthy."

While asking a lover to test for transmittable diseases may not seem sexy, seeing that the test results are negative calls for a sexual celebration! Testing for STDs together, like communicating about sexual limits in general, is a sign of mutual trust and respect. Once you and your partner are both certain that you are disease free, honor the results of the blood tests by avoiding the exchange of fluids with anyone else. Respect and protect each other at all times. Nothing makes for hotter sex than safety.

Learning to share in the pleasures of the Paradise Found Sexual Ceremony is likely to shed valuable light on the essence of your sexual identity as well as your selfhood. To delve deeper into the sexual realm is to delve deeper into the inner self. As joyful as this should be, it may be a difficult, if not painful, experience for some. Safer sex thus also means providing for emotional protection, in case the sexual experience incites emotions that go beyond those that we commonly associate with pleasure.

Unfortunately, an enormous percentage of us were, either deliberately or inadvertently, sexually repressed or even traumatized. Neglect, abuse, violence, and abandonment are not uncommon in childhood or in the lives of sexually mature adults; repercussions from traumatic events should not be ignored. If there are issues that you cannot confront alone or with your partner, do not hesitate to seek professional assistance from a therapist or psychologist.

Though we cannot control or change our past, we can guide and shape our future by working to recognize, rather than repress, the negative influences that sexual trauma, as well as social conditioning, can impose. By unraveling constrictive emotional knots, we begin to take our sexual evolution back into our own hands. By discerning the limits that bind our freedom of sexual expression, we may gradually surmount them and begin to follow our desires without inhibition, in harmony with our needs and fantasies. Learning, accepting, and, if necessary, healing our sexual personae are crucial for being able to share the potentially transcendental powers of sex as well as for overall happiness and well-being.

LIKING, SWIPING, AND HOOKING UP: THE TWENTY-FIRST-CENTURY DATING GAME

There are many winding paths to the Paradise Found Sexual Ceremony, and it would be remiss not to give a nod to the impact on our sexuality—and the possibilities to explore it—that the digital age provides. Looking for love or for the next "hook-up" is now just a like, swipe, and click away. We are hooking up and dating more frequently, with a pool of potential lovers that has multiplied by hundreds, if not thousands. The human brain is "wired" to evolve and elaborate relationships with approximately three hundred people—from family members, friends, and colleagues to lovers—over the course of a lifetime. Today we can virtually meet three hundred people and more in one day, so the evolution of the human race is definitely getting a revolutionary digital kick!

This expansive sense of possibility, a reality for those who tap into it, may prompt frightened doomsayers to prophesize the crumbling of civilization, but ultimately, online dating is not altering our need for intimacy or love nor is it changing the way that we have sex. No matter how technologically advanced we humans become, sexual attraction remains under chemistry's animalistic sway. What is changing, however, are our dating rituals as well as our perceptions of the parameters of relationships.

Whether or not you personally nurture your primal instinct by connecting online—and liking, chatting, hearting, and swiping prospective mates into intimacy—you most certainly know someone who has found dates, sex, or even love thanks to the Internet.

Liberté, Équalité, Fraternité
Sexual desire and, at least subconsciously, the desire to find love, have been the prime motivators for humans throughout history and remain so during the digital age. Some of us use online dating platforms to seek a soulmate with whom to build a strong and durable relationship, while others "hook up" for casual, anonymous sex using the accelerated heartbeat of mobile dating applications. With the invention of the smartphone and mobile dating applications, the world has become not only our mobile office but also our boudoir. Matchmaking algorithms, detailed personal profiles, social media engagement, and geolocators that indicate the proximity of potential dates and hook-ups are the strategies of the digital dating game. Depending on how you play it, your next date or one-night stand could be sitting in the bar next door. Your evening at home alone is just a few swipes and a chat away from the company of a more-than-friendly neighbor who is in the mood to "watch Netflix and chill." Whether you are planning to "hook up" for casual sex or hoping to find a like-minded individual with whom to cultivate meaningful bonds, the goal of the dating game should positively be pleasure.

Positive dating experiences on the Internet are not a myth: a 2014 online dating survey revealed that 79 percent of Internet daters had a positive experience. Of those surveyed, a full 34 percent had found a significant partner, compared to surveyed singles who were not dating online, of whom only 3 percent had found their personal "match." Technology is truly contributing to the vitality of our sex lives, our love lives, and, last but not least, to the building of enduring relationships. This is encouraging news, as the ability to build healthy intimate bonds is a measure of our emotional and mental well-being.

And the so-called generational digital divide is also closing: while younger, computer-savvy generations find new friends and lovers on the Internet just as naturally as they work, shop, and play on it, those who grew up before WiFi became a word have gradually joined them, encouraged by the happy, adventurous, and successful stories of online daters. Also the notion that women who date online are "desperate"—a myth rooted in gender bias—or anyone who uses digital matchmaking services is a "loser" is thankfully disappearing.

In fact, the Internet is giving digital daters, no matter their gender or sexual orientation, a powerful sense of sexual liberation as well a radical amplification of their chances to meet sexually compatible individuals and significant others beyond established social circuits. Digital dating is also helping to "normalize" sexual behaviors that were once considered unacceptable. Openly seeking a BDSM playmate and organizing a threesome (or a moresome) for the sake of no-strings-attached pleasure has never been easier, more openly public, or as legally protected as it is today. This is especially relevant and liberating for the LGBTQIA+ community, who until recently was obliged to hook up undercover in LGBTQIA+-specific venues or in potentially dangerous public places like city parks and parking lots.

Online dating also equalizes gender-biased relationship rituals; single women are taking advantage of the newfound freedom to play the dating game as openly as heterosexual males have been playing it for centuries. The days when women who "made the first move" were stigmatized as "easy" or "loose" are coming to an end.

Even those who practice polyamory are taking advantage of the freedom and opportunities provided by the Internet to extend their multiple bonds. Consolidated polyamorist families are composed of consenting adults who are openly committed to each other and who agree to exercise honest open communication at all times. Honesty marks the difference between polyamory and adultery or infidelity, which is, of course, also thriving online.

Today's gardens of earthly delight have truly become a virtual playground: simply name your desire, and you can probably fulfill it online.

From Stranger to Lover
No matter how you date or look for love, consider sex to be more than a banal, consumeristic "product." During sex, our peripersonal space—the immediate space surrounding our body that is also described by neurologists as the "second skin"—merges and blends with that of our partner(s). The potent effect of this merging of energy is radically intensified when penetration is not off-limits. The quality of our sexual exchanges can be the factor that determines whether relationships evolve into more significant and enduring ones (or not).

Consider your intimate relationships as journeys, not pit stops, and you will reap and share in infinitely greater pleasure. The crescendo of physical, emotional, and spiritual pleasure experienced by those who are genuinely attracted to each other and who take the time to get to know one another better in the context of a sexual ceremony is impossible to experience with a total stranger. There are two simple reasons for this: trust and time.

Whether you date on- or offline, the better you get to know

someone, the more you can trust them and the more likely it is that your sexual exchanges will be positive and increasingly pleasurable. Lack of trust in one's partner is the main reason that "fast" PGO sex is usually at the top of the hooking-up menu (unless you are using a BDSM app to connect with like-minded individuals who don't solely seek the quick release of genitally oriented sexual tension). Heterosexual women tend to be the least satisfied when it comes to mobile hooking up; this is not surprising, considering that "fast" sex is not the route to enhanced female pleasure. It takes more than one night to know anyone well enough to trust them and to "let go," body and soul, into the greater pleasures that the sexual and sensual realms have to offer. Sexual abandon is integral to deep and all-encompassing sexual satisfaction, and trust, its facilitator, belongs to any truly satisfying sexual encounter. The importance of trust is all the more relevant when lovers privilege the powerful tools and techniques of full-body stimulation.

The good news is that everyone we get to know better was once a stranger to our hearts. Experience has taught me this: if you find yourself genuinely attracted to a stranger, no matter how you may have met this person, he or she won't remain a stranger for long if the connection between you is mutual. Mutual attraction is a rare seed that can be cultivated beyond what might have been intended to be a fleeting one-night stand. So if the sparks of desire fly between you and your partner, don't be jaded. Don't dismiss. Keep your body, mind, and spirit open to finding more than a bon coup, as the French say.

Only one in one hundred virtual connections may result in an offline mutual attraction—so be prepared to dedicate time to the dating game. Quantity cannot replace quality when it comes to sex, so if you wish to find a partner with whom to explore and experience the all-encompassing levels of sexual satisfaction that are integral to the Paradise Found Sexual Ceremony, be patient and point your online dating strategy toward dating, not hooking up.

Prepare Yourself for the Virtual Plunge
Before signing into a dating platform or downloading a mobile dating app onto your phone, ask yourself: What am I looking for? How do I best portray myself in order to increase the possibility of obtaining what I am looking for? And, most importantly, before you have initiated a real face-to-face date, how can my offline dating boundaries facilitate my search?

People who know what they want out of life are more likely to get it than those who just "go with the flow." The more honest you are with yourself, the more likely it is that you will find what you seek in the virtual sea of love, lust, and desire. Mystery, confusion, dishonesty, and fakery abound in this world, so do the world and yourself a favor: Be real. Be honest. Be yourself!

But sometimes we are our own worst enemies: statistics reveal that what we cruise, like, and swipe right is often the opposite of what we say, or believe, we want. Our subconscious does indeed exert a powerful hold on our happiness! Seeking to understand yourself through yoga or meditation, or with the help of a psychologist, if you feel the necessity, will help to harmonize conscious and subconscious desires. Unrealistic expectations also sabotage many a search for sex and love. Dating platforms and apps claim they will find your "perfect match" or your "soulmate." The "perfect" lover is an age-old fairy tale that continues to be celebrated by Hollywood, literature, the media, and religion today. But enduring relationships are hinged on tolerance and patience as much as they are on love and respect. Our funny quirks and little imperfections that set us apart also bring us together, so they should be celebrated, not denigrated.

Unrealistic expectations of ourselves and others cause us to doubt our own potential or hop from one person to another on a frustratingly impossible quest for perfection. Go into the online dating game with a sense of fun, universal love, and adventure—and most importantly, prioritize shared pleasure, not perfection. You will certainly meet several worthy ceremonial partners and possibly even a serious significant other if you do. Relationships cannot be forced into predetermined shapes. Instead, appreciate the uniqueness of each intimate journey that you take and remember that the outcome of every connection that you make, on- or offline, will always be determined by one very critical and uncontrollable factor: chemistry. Algorithms cannot generate that mysterious spark. All algorithms and geolocators can do is enhance the possibility that the fires of desire will be ignited.

Stress Less, Feel More!
With seemingly infinite choices, digital dating sends some users into synaptic overload. You may be one of those users who have hundreds or even thousands of potential connections smoldering in your "vault," or you may have been swept into a full-blown dating or hooking-up spree that leaves you neglecting your own needs offline. Emotional confusion and stress may occur—or for some a bodily and emotional numbness—if you hook up on a regular basis exclusively for anonymous sex, with no real consideration for or interest in the individual lying naked next you beyond a quick casual hook-up.

It's true that you might thrive on engaging in multiple encounters and the feeling of being "liked" or "swiped right." You promise you'll start out responsibly, maintaining sensible boundaries like meeting strangers in public and always using a condom, but all too easily waning excitement can lead to boredom and cavalier behavior, which inevitably breeds a dissatisfaction that pushes the boundaries toward riskier behavior. Such a cycle can result in a physical and emotional numbness; a sort of sexual dependence can ensue.

The constant search for casual no-strings-attached sexual companionship, like the impossible quest for the perfect partner, consumes time and energy. If, instead of finding pleasure in the digital dating game, you find yourself stressing out or feeling emotionally spent or numb, go offline and spend time with people who care about you, even if sex is not on the menu. After all, we need more than just sex to be happy. We need to feel connected. We want to feel love.

Ultimately, sex should make us feel good and if you are not satisfied take it as a sign. Let your personal experiences, including the good and the bad, be your best lessons. Avoid self-loathing and remain true to yourself. There are people out there in this big world who will love you for who you really are.

Painting Your Digital Portrait
If, as the saying goes, a picture is worth a thousand words, then your profile says almost everything about you. The way you fill out your profile will affect how the path of your online dating experience will wend. Be as honest as possible, so the matchmaking algorithms will filter out people who have nothing in common with you, saving your precious time and energy—two of the great luxuries of the twenty-first century.

Do fellow online daters a courtesy and post a recent photograph of yourself (not your best buddy, a group shot, one with your ex-girlfriend, or your pet). Your favorite picture, taken a few years ago when you were decisively younger, more fit, and in what you consider to be your "prime" is also not acceptable unless you haven't really changed a bit. I have heard too many stories of disappointment from people who found themselves sitting in front of an online date who looked nothing at all like his or her profile picture. Filling out a profile or status is not mandatory on most dating services, but sharing information about yourself will generate more traffic and better matches. Making your intentions clear in your status will also help you clarify your own motivations. The more concise and captivating your message, the more likely you are to attract someone who might intrigue you.

Profile pictures and statuses ideally reveal our intentions: people who seek stable relationships will have a very different approach to their online presentation than those who are seeking anonymous, no-strings-attached, one-night stands. (A hook-up-weary friend once told me that he was "finished with connecting with torsos or other body parts"!) If you want more than fast, casual sex, present yourself as more than an available body. Share images that reflect your true self and the world that you live in along with words that complement your honest search. Being honest to yourself and fellow humans is crucial to the art of living.

In turn, when you are looking at others' profiles, contemplate the pictures carefully: as the saying goes, our eyes are the windows to our souls, so learn to read the eyes as well as the body language of the people you connect with. Scan the wording of the profile to see if it complements the message of the portrait. Be aware of acronyms like "H&H" (high and horny) or "P&P" (party and play); casual sex mixed with hard drugs or alcohol—and with a stranger— is a dangerous cocktail indeed. While people have inhibitions about sex and feel the need to relax or enhance their experience with drugs and alcohol, note that excessive intoxication or inebriation skews our perceptions and inhibits the flow of our bodies' natural "love drugs," not to mention our sense of sexual satisfaction. Protect yourself by learning to read between the lines of a profile to dis- cover—and discard—incompatible matches.

It is true that once you have uploaded your profile picture and turned on the geolocator, the sheer quantity of people cruising the virtual scene will send a rush of hopeful excitement through your veins. And it won't take long before you find yourself at ease with the process of uninhibitedly swiping potential lovers right (into)—or left (out of)—your virtual realm of sexual possibility. Of course, in the real world, treating other humans as summarily and ruthlessly as this would be, at best, rude, and at worst, potentially dangerous. But this is how online relationships begin. Just remember people are not products, even though they, like any online dater (including you), have packaged and presented themselves to appeal. The people that you accept into your "vault" are human beings just like you: brave and vulnerable.

Even Wallflowers Bloom Online!
You have made your first "like" and behold, you are "liked" back. Having taken the place of traditional courting rituals, chatting online serves to make one pleasure-vital decision: to meet or not to meet? The screen—in both acting as a kind of safety net and providing a fun, gamelike quality to online interactions with potential dates or hook-ups—coaxes us to flirt and share very personal information about ourselves with total strangers (and much more readily than we would ever be inclined to exchange offline and in person). Like the love notes of days gone by, chatting about our desires, needs, and sex in general stimulates the pleasure center of our brains. Gradually increasing the erotic and graphic sexual communication is a potent kind of foreplay that will prompt the flow of the body's feel-good hormones like oxytocin. While it is easy to allow erotic communication to escalate into something more graphic, don't mislead strangers with heavy sexting if your intention is to stay at home in bed. Fluffing people further than you are willing and ready to go is not appreciated on- or offline.

Whether you are looking for anonymous sex or a soulmate, respect and treat others as you wish to be treated. Individuals who overstep your online limits will almost certainly continue to do so if you decide to give them your precious time offline. Abusive language and abusive behavior generally go hand and hand, so "unlike" individuals whose standards do not match your needs, desires, and values. Remember that you are not ever obliged to proceed with any interaction, online or offline.

As you chat, don't be shy about broaching topics that are personal yet important to discuss before two strangers get intimate: the use of condoms; health issues, such as STDs; relationship status; the interest in full-body stimulation rather than "fast" PGO sex; the use of drugs and alcohol—these and more should be up for discussion. Nevertheless, many people do not tell the truth about what they want, who they are, or even their age and occupation and other pertinent personal details. The Internet is virtually writhing with imposters and while we can't force others to be honest, passing the virtual chemistry test requires that you feel safe. You will know when it's time to get offline and meet your match in person.

Flirt with Your Date, Not with Disaster
Experienced players know that "sexting" can turn the heat up high, but the virtual connection will lose traction quickly if both users don't agree to meet in the real world fairly swiftly. If you intend to hook up with the aroused stranger that is dangling from your sizzling-hot hook as soon as you hang up, it is important to have established a few extra personal boundaries, as well as take the safer-sex precautions discussed in the prior section of The Boudoir Bible.

Man, woman, transgender, gay, straight, or bi—and no matter what you are looking for in life—establishing boundaries and sticking to them (until you know someone well enough to feel genuinely safe in pushing them) can make the difference between a life well lived and a life full of complications and regrets. And, as equalizing and liberating as online dating may seem, there are risks that women who date online undergo that men do not, as statistics from both the United States and UK highlight in dating a stranger, with the victims of 85 percent of all online first-date rapes being women.

Unlike traditional blind dates, which are arranged by trusted friends or family members, the people with whom you virtually connect are most often not part of your offline social network. Via chatting, as I've explained, you can learn a little more about your potential date or hook-up before meeting in person, but advice for safer, more pleasurable meetings follow:

- Especially if you are a woman, why not take one more virtual communication step before fixing a time and place to meet your online date? Hearing his or her voice will tell you a lot about that person, but a virtual face-to-face is even better: it will also help to ensure that a potential in-person meeting will not be a disappointing waste of either player's precious time.

- Regardless of your gender, the following should be considered an unbending rule for anyone playing the digital dating game: Get to know your date in a neutral and public location where there is no risk of finding yourself totally alone. If your date is really worth your precious time, much less your precious body, he or she will be more than happy to meet you in public. If your date insists otherwise, look for another date. And it must be said: Going to the home of a stranger or asking him or her to come to yours for a first date is as dangerous as providing your home address. (And getting into the car of a total stranger on a first date is out of the question.) Playing safe is a basic courtesy to yourself and those who love you.

- Being sober is crucial to our ability to read people, not to mention our sexual satisfaction. If you opt to go to a restaurant or a bar, commit to one (slow) drink and pay for your own dinner or drink to avoid the situation in which the other person (or you) feels you need to return "the favor." Go dutch and get home safely.

- Never turn your phone off during the date but as a courtesy do turn the sound off so that you and your date are not distracted by push alerts and calls.

- Let a friend know your plans before you go on a date, especially if you plan on having sex. Organizing a security text or call is easy and effective—consider it as a sort of safety belt when you are in the mood to hook up. Set an alarm so you don't forget to make the call or send that text. As an extra precaution, send the online information about your date or hook-up to a trusted friend as well as the address of where you will be. Take your preestablished security communication seriously; don't make people who care about you worry. If it is your friend's duty to call or text you and he or she doesn't manage to reach you after several attempts, then your friend should call the police.

- Note that not all countries use or perceive the use of online dating equally—if digital dating is considered illegal in the country where you are traveling, simply do not partake.

- And a word on the safety of others: If you happen across someone whom you suspect to be a minor while cruising online, do the responsible thing: tell him or her to get off the app or dating platform. Dating apps are designed for sexually mature adults. It is our duty to protect minors who are unknowingly putting themselves in danger. Internet governance bodies give little to no consideration to children's rights.

The Digital Embrace
Since the turn of the twenty-first century, I have been advising individuals who have felt "stuck" in abstinence to break out of their

sexless shells and take advantage of the Internet to find new lovers, ceremonial partners, and, potentially, significant others. I also encourage any of you, my readers, who are experiencing similar frustrations, to dedicate some time to research the digital dating options that might best suit your needs and to sign in to the possibility of revitalizing your sex life, and maybe much more, online. There could not be a more obvious nor natural evolution of our courting rituals, considering that we live in a society that is not only striving for sexual freedom and equality but also thriving on technology. Embrace online dating as a service and an amazing tool, as well as an opportunity to connect ever more deeply with yourself and a potential ceremonial partner. The gates of Paradise await!

CHAPTER 1

————o————

THE ANATOMY OF DESIRE:
A COMPARATIVE APPROACH

Our bodies are our gardens, to the which our wills are gardeners.

— Iago, *Othello*, William Shakespeare

THE MALE AND FEMALE genitals are the center of the human body's vast garden of sensual delights, and our fascination with them is innate. But our perception of the genitals (and the body as a whole) is still shaped by pleasure-inhibiting myths and misconceptions that were founded on Judeo-Christian morals.

The fathers of Western philosophy can be considered instigators of the destructive mind-body dichotomy that led to the denigration of humanity's physical being. It began with Plato (427–347 B.C.) and his seminal dialogue *Phaedo*, wherein the dialectician Socrates, awaiting his execution, considers the chasm between the temporal body and the immortal soul. Aristotle (384–322 B.C.), the foremost student of Plato, furthered this point of view on the relationship of mind to body, developing a position on the relationship of male to female that Judeo-Christian authorities would later solidify into dogma.

Aristotle placed great emphasis upon the differences between the genders, which included the male and female reproductive systems. Considering man to be whole, or intact, he thought of women as little more than "mutilated" and "deformed" males, going so far as to maintain that the male gender was entirely responsible for the creation of life. He limited women's role in procreation to the housing of homunculi, the miniature, preformed individuals he believed to be stored in the male testicles. The uterus was only a convenient vessel in which the miraculous, creative powers of man were carried to term.

It was not until the end of the seventeenth century that this construction would be scientifically challenged. In 1672, with the help of a rudimentary microscope, Dutch physician Reinier de Graaf discovered what he thought to be eggs (but were actually the follicles on the ovaries, in which the ova grow). Five years later, Antonie van Leeuwenhoek, the Dutch microscopist and a student of de Graaf, discovered spermatozoa. But the critical role of woman in the procreative process would not be scientifically proven until 1879, when the Swiss physician and zoologist Hermann Fol finally observed the entry of a sperm into an egg. Although his research was conducted with sea urchins, it served to prove that males and females had equally important roles in the procreative process. This led to the conclusion that women were not nearly as incomplete or pro-creatively passive as early philosophical authorities had taught. All the same, men continued to be considered superior to their female counterparts, both sexually and in virtually every aspect of human existence beyond the domestic domain until the revolutionary 1960s.

It was not until the second half of the relatively enlightened twentieth century that researchers would scientifically prove that sexual satisfaction is not determined by gender, that woman's ability to experience heightened degrees of sexual pleasure is in no way inferior to that of their male counterparts, and that the male and female genitals are not nearly as different as they appear to be on the surface.

In spite of the past fifty years of "liberation," the magical source of the sexual vibration is still shrouded in shame and misunderstanding. To dismantle pleasure-inhibiting myths and misconceptions and eventually unveil the extent of our bodies' capacity to provide pleasure, a better understanding of what I call "the anatomy of desire" must be acquired.

X + X = X + Y: THE ANATOMY EQUATION

First, let's put our most apparent differences into perspective by taking a closer look at the formative stages of human life. As we all learned in biology class at school, the combination of two X chromosomes determines the female gender, while that of the X and Y chromosomes results in the male sex. But what our teachers failed to tell us is that, from a biological point of view, we all start out as same-sexed creatures. Gender differentiation does not occur until the eighth week of gestation. When a fetus is genetically determined to be male, at that time it is showered with gender-differentiating hormones such as testosterone. This same hormonal shower serves as a signal for Mother Nature to "sew up" what would otherwise continue to develop into the female genitals, resulting in a pouch of skin—the scrotum—that is joined in the middle by what looks like a seam.

The female fetus does not receive a similar shower of estrogen, as the role of that hormone does not come fully into play until girls reach puberty, at which time estrogen surges, helping to build the breasts and the hips of a budding woman and prompting her monthly menstrual cycle.

Male or female, the genitals are fully formed by the sixteenth week of gestation, and while the final results appear distinctly different from an anatomical point of view, the male and female genitals are composed of analogous components that share similar forms and functions. By exploring our similarities, rather than emphasizing our differences, we can begin to reevaluate the merits of our differences and evolve as more informed and confident sexual equals.

In the sections that follow, please refer to the comparative anatomical illustrations of the male and female genitals on plates II–III, pages 66-67, which highlight our similarities, making for a more comprehensive understanding of sexual anatomy and physiology.

The Penis at Rest
From an early age, a boy cannot help but be familiar with the streamlined architecture of his penis, composed of the shaft, the glans, called the head, and the scrotum. The shaft, extending from within the body, between the scrotum and the anus, to the glans, which crowns the penis, defines this organ's length and breadth. The glans, the most sensitive area of the male body, is protected (in uncircumcised men) when the penis is not erect by a double layer of retractable skin known as the prepuce, or foreskin. The foreskin is connected to the frenulum, the tissue connected to the V-shaped notch in the glans on the underside of the penis. The removal of the foreskin via circumcision exposes the frenulum and the glans in its entirety, even when the penis is at rest.

The scrotal sac, with its primordial seam, is positioned approximately two-thirds down the length of the shaft. Within the sac are carried the testicles, or gonads, where spermatozoa, the vital seed of the male sex, and other hormones are produced and stored. (Neither sperm nor ejaculate fluid is generated until the male's puberty.) The only opening in the penis is at its tip. Nicknamed the U-spot in the 1980s, the urethral opening releases both urine from the bladder and semen from the male reproductive tract. The glands that generate the ejaculate fluid are explored later in this chapter.

The Matrix and the Crown Jewel
The female genitals—with their more internal, less "obvious" design

than the male genitals—tend to be misunderstood, in part because of the dire state of modern-day sex education. Take, for example, the American system of sex education programming, which has long been a pawn in a political game between religious conservatives and liberal groups. As late as the 1960s, sex education programs were not mandatory, and schools that opted to offer sex education were obliged to limit the subject matter to sexual anatomy, disease, and reproduction. Even during the first decade of the twenty-first century, during the Bush administration, state funding was denied to any public school that did not teach "abstinence only" sex education, although studies have proven that this kind of focus does nothing to prevent teen pregnancy or halt the spread of sexually transmitted diseases. And, unfortunately, while funding for comprehensive teen pregnancy prevention has improved under the Obama administration, the taboo-ridden topics of sexual well-being and satisfaction are still off-limits within the classroom.

And so it is little wonder that the female genitals continue to inspire misunderstanding, as well as terminological confusion. The word "vagina," for example, is all too often incorrectly used to describe the female genitals as a whole. I recently cringed over and over again while reading an Eve Ensler–inspired article entitled "The Vagina Dialogues" in a popular women's magazine. Among other absurdities, the dyeing, shaving, and waxing of the vagina are mentioned. (*Ouch!*) When sex education truly becomes educational, the term "vagina" will be used to indicate the vaginal canal alone, not the female genitals as a whole. The term *vulva*, Latin for "wrapping," or "matrix," should be used to correctly indicate the visible portion of the female genitals, and, more precisely, the visible elements of the clitoral system. The etymology of *vulva* suggests that the ancient Romans, noted masters of the arts of erotic loving, were well aware of the gifts that lie within its organic, flowerlike form.

Women (and men) are rarely encouraged to simply observe

and explore the female genitals, and many young girls reach sexual maturity without ever having looked at the marvel that lies between their legs. If you are a woman and have never viewed your own vulva, use a mirror to familiarize yourself with each visible element of your genitals, referring also to plate II, page 66. If you are a man and your partner is a woman, share in the joy that such an exploration can yield. Shedding deep-rooted genital taboos and guilt is crucial to our ability to partake of the pleasures that our genitals are designed to provide.

The crown jewel of the vulva is the female glans, more commonly known as the clitoris. The clitoris, which expands inward rather than outward as the penis does, is deceivingly small. However, when the clitoral system, which is actually composed of eighteen different elements, is considered in its entirety, it is comparable in size to the male genital structure.

Like the male glans, the female glans is composed of erectile tissues that become turgid during sexual arousal. The clitoris contains more nerve endings than any other area of the female or male body, and, remarkably, it is the only component of the human anatomy whose sole function is to provide sexual pleasure.

The inner lips, or labia minora, of the vagina, framing its entryway, converge just below the pubic mound to form the clitoral hood and the bridle. The clitoral hood corresponds to the foreskin in males, and it represents the greatest visual similarity between the male and female genitals—when the penis is at rest and if the foreskin has been left intact. Like the foreskin, the clitoral hood protects the glans. The bridle, framing the clitoris, corresponds to the frenulum in males. It is similarly represented by a distinctive upside-down V shape. In both men and women, the frenulum constitutes a very sensitive area of the body.

The female urethral opening (U-spot), the smallest orifice in the vulva's panorama, is capable of providing extremely pleasurable

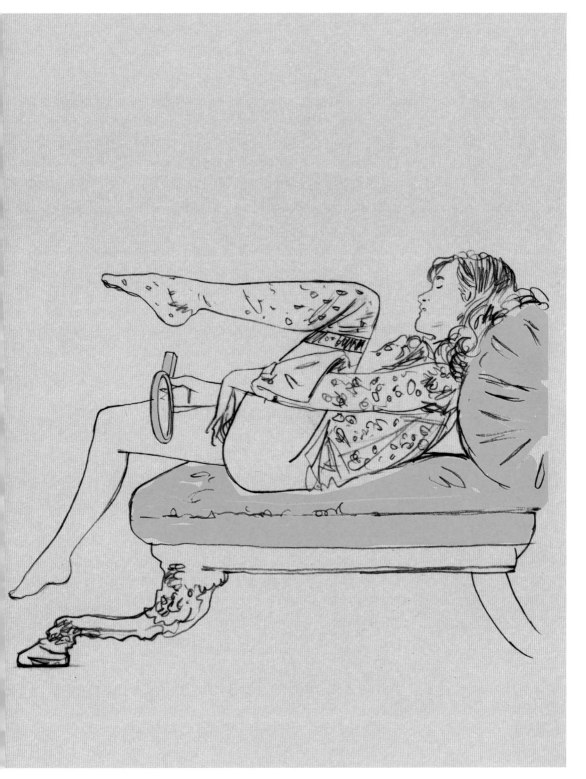

PLATE I RITUAL MASTURBATION SESSION WITH MIRROR

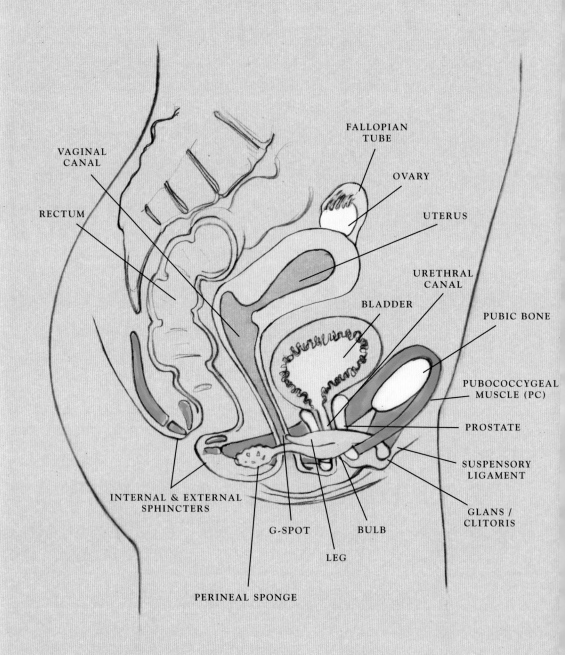

FALLOPIAN TUBE

OVARY

UTERUS

VAGINAL CANAL

RECTUM

URETHRAL CANAL

BLADDER

PUBIC BONE

PUBOCOCCYGEAL MUSCLE (PC)

PROSTATE

SUSPENSORY LIGAMENT

INTERNAL & EXTERNAL SPHINCTERS

GLANS / CLITORIS

G-SPOT

BULB

LEG

PERINEAL SPONGE

PLATE II THE FEMALE GENITALS: SIDE VIEW

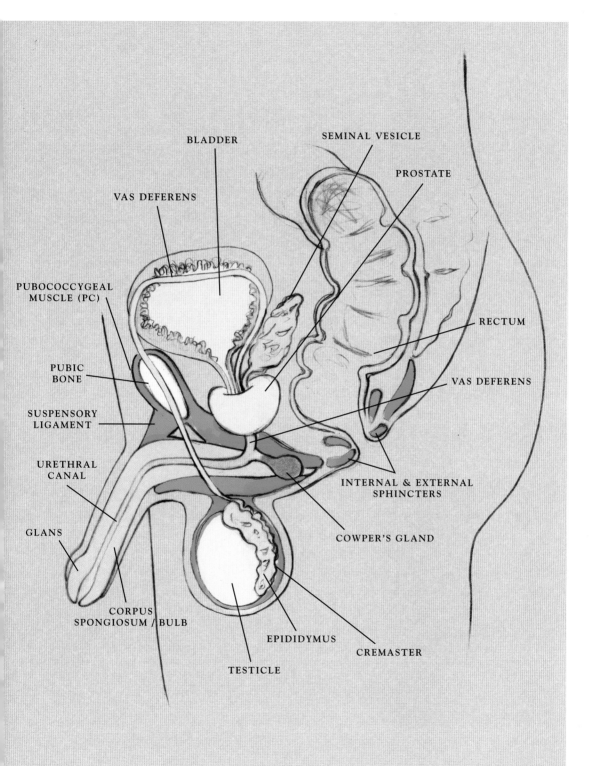

PLATE III THE MALE GENITALS: SIDE VIEW

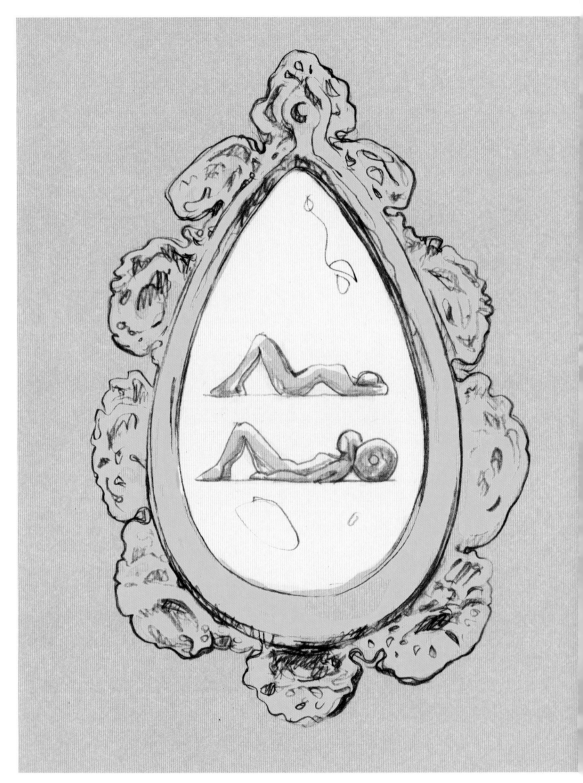

PLATE IV THE HYSTERICAL ARCH AND ITS INVERSION

sensations, just as the glans does for men, especially when stimulated orally. The entryway to the vaginal canal is the largest opening in the vulva. Visible remnants of the hymen, the fine membrane that closes the entryway to the vaginal canal from birth to adolescence, may be seen from the opening of the vaginal canal. The integrity of the hymen was considered proof of female virginity, but unjustly so, as the hymen can erode or be broken long before a penis—or anything else, for that matter—penetrates the vaginal opening. The hymen is considered part of the clitoral system, as is the fourchette, the area of skin that lies directly behind the opening of the vagina.

As predominant as they are in the female genital geography, the fleshy outer lips of the vulva, known as the labia majora, are not considered part of the clitoral system. From an anatomical point of comparison, the labia majora correspond to the male scrotum, but they obviously do not serve the same function.

Unless you make use of a speculum, you will not be able to see inside the vaginal canal, but you can manually explore the entryway and the soft inner walls of the vagina. Use your middle finger to locate the pronounced, firm, miniature-doughnut-like shape of the cervix at the very end of the vaginal canal. From a spermatozoon's perspective, the cervix is the portal to the uterus, and for an unborn baby, it represents the exit from the mother's body into the outside world. The uterus is the hearth, as it were, of the female reproductive system, and it is the only major component of the female genital geography that does not have a parallel with the male genitals. The ovaries, which are situated on the upper left and right sides of the uterus, correspond to the testicles in men.

The ova are housed in the ovaries, which are each attended by a Fallopian tube. Once a month, during the process of ovulation, one of the tubes transports what is usually a single ovum into the uterus. Whether or not this egg encounters a vital spermatozoon and thus sparks the miraculous creative process of life is—and should remain—a private decision. That heterosexual couples are no longer obliged to carry the burden of unplanned conception from their shared sexual pleasures should not be taken for granted.

THE ERECTION: A SHARED DELIGHT

The interior aspects of both the male and female reproductive system are made up of erectile tissues, muscles, glands, and an intricate map of nerves, veins, and blood vessels. Both male and female genitals, when sexually stimulated, gradually dilate and become turgid as the veins and blood vessels in the erectile tissues are engorged with blood.

The male erection is essentially a hydraulic phenomenon that occurs in the columns of the corpora cavernosa and the corpus spongiosum, also known as the bulb. As blood fills the arteries and vascular channels and the penis becomes erect, muscles compress these spongy masses of tissue, preventing blood from draining back into the body.

The corpus spongiosum corresponds to the twin vestibular bulbs in females, which are also composed of spongy erectile tissues. Because the vestibular bulbs, which represent one of the densest portions of the clitoral system, lie inside the female body, on either side of the vaginal canal, physical alterations in an aroused woman's genitals are less obvious than those that occur in the penis.

The vestibular bulbs respond to sexual stimulation in a similar fashion to the male's spongy tissues, but as the vestibular bulbs swell with blood, the walls of the vaginal canal dilate and expand inward rather than outward. The changes that take place can be imagined as a sort of internal erection and can be felt with the fingertips or the sensitive tip of the penis.

Over extended periods of stimulation, the entire clitoral system will expand and cause visible transformations to occur outside the body as well. The vulva will swell with pleasure, and the clitoris will assume a position pointing outward and upward, due to the erection of the clitoral shaft, located most easily during arousal by pressing the clitoris in and slightly upward, toward the pubic mound.

Apply pressure to either side of the clitoris (again, ideally during arousal), and you will notice that the shaft divides, creating the clitoral legs, or crura. The crura flare out from the clitoral shaft and run between the inner and outer lips, permitting women to experience clitoral pleasures without actually making direct contact with the tender button itself.

The clitoral erection is accompanied by the phenomenon of self-lubrication. Two small round glands, known as the Bartholin's glands, are located on either side of the entryway to the vagina. The duct of each gland emits a slippery secretion on the surface of the vulva. The activity of the Bartholin's ducts, along with the self-lubrication of the vagina, indicates heightened sexual arousal in most women. As these titillating phenomena take place, the vulva flushes darker shades of red, pink, purple, or black, depending on skin tone. A similar display of sexual excitement also occurs in men. All such visible transformations are subtle signals of enhanced sensitivity and receptivity to touch. During the Paradise Found Sexual Ceremony, when lovers enjoy prolonged periods of worshiping one another, these subtle signals of heightened sexual arousal become increasingly evident.

THE FOUNTAINHEAD OF EMISSION

This leads us to the most obvious signal of heightened sexual arousal, the phenomenon of ejaculation, which directly correlates to the prostate gland. The male prostate gland is a spongy network of erectile tissues with a distinct chestnut-like shape that surrounds the base of the urethra. Its position in the body—adjacent to the wall of the rectum, approximately 3 inches (7.5 centimeters) inside the anus—is the main reason the male prostate gland remains shrouded in mystery and shame. Many heterosexual men are not "anal friendly" and commonly refrain from exploring the pleasures of prostate stimulation for fear of being considered or even "turning into" a homosexual. The only way to locate or stimulate the male prostate gland directly is to hurdle the taboo of anal penetration. Prostate stimulation should be enjoyed as a natural source of heightened pleasure, no matter one's sexual orientation. The gland and its relation to anal health and pleasure is explored further in the chapter "The Anthems of Anal Sex: From Hygiene to Heavenly Pleasures."

From a purely clinical point of view, the male prostate gland produces, stores, and emits a clear alkaline substance that makes up part of the ejaculate fluid that is commonly called semen. Male prostate fluid is known to guarantee favorable procreative conditions by protecting the sperm as they travel toward the outside world. It also gives semen its characteristic viscosity and color.

The fact that women have an organ that corresponds to the male prostate as well as the capacity to produce and emit ejaculate fluid has been long repressed, shunned, and even denied. But pre-Judeo-Christian art, architecture, literature, and artifacts indicate that the phenomenon of female ejaculation was once considered a natural and integrated—if not sacred—aspect of female pleasure. It was not until the 1970s that sex researchers began to study this organ and its functions more seriously.

By 1981, the female counterpart of the male prostate was finally scientifically proven to exist, and it was given its first name—the urethral sponge—by Carol Downer, the founder of the Federation of Feminist Women's Health Centers (FFWHC) and her colleagues. But it was not until 2001 that the Federative Committee on Anatomical Terminology finally gave the organ its official name: the female prostate.

Like the male prostate, the female prostate is composed of a network of erectile tissues, ducts, and paraurethral glands that surround the base of the urethral canal. Though the female prostate is smaller and more elongated in comparison to the male prostate gland, it makes up for its size by being composed of nearly three times the number of glands and ducts. The primary function of the female prostate is similar to that of its male counterpart—that of manufacturing, storing, and emitting ejaculate fluid. The chemical composition of this fluid is alkaline, just like that produced in the male prostate. The largest gland associated with the female prostate is the Skene's gland, located on either side of the urethral opening. It works with numerous other glands that lie deeper inside the spongy structure to produce this fluid.

The most tangible manifestation of the female prostate is a slightly raised, irregular, almond-shaped mass of erectile tissue located on the upper anterior (front) wall of the vaginal canal, approximately ½ inch to 2 inches (2 to 5 centimeters) from the vaginal opening. It is more commonly known today as the infamous and ever-so-generous G-spot. The G-spot is the crown of the female prostate, the root of the clitoral system, and the key to female emission. It was given its name by the sex researchers Beverly Whipple and John D. Perry in honor of Dr. Ernst Grafenberg, who had, already by 1950, associated the sensitive spot with enhanced female pleasure.

"JUST USE YOUR FINGERS!"

In 2008, BBC.com posted an article entitled "The Female G-spot 'Can Be Detected,'" reporting that an Italian scientist had made the discovery with ultrasound. I remember saying out loud to myself, "You don't need an ultrasound to find it, Sherlock—just use your fingers!" I bookmarked the article and forgot about it until almost exactly two years later, when my e-mail in-box overflowed with messages from friends, colleagues, and clients who wanted to call my attention to an article posted by the same source that was entitled "The G-Spot 'Doesn't Appear to Exist,' Say Researchers."

The journalist had failed to cite any details of the clinical research that had proven the contrary thirty years prior, but they did contact Dr. Beverly Whipple, a major figure in the research.

Whipple defended the cause of the G-spot, the existence of which she had worked so hard to prove, by stating that the research in question, which was performed only on sets of twins, was "flawed." She also said that it "discounted the experiences of lesbian or bisexual women and failed to consider the effects of having different sexual partners with different love-making techniques." I felt that it would have been appropriate if she had finished her statement with "Amen," or, rather, "Awomen!"

Both my research and my personal experience allowed me to reassure the women who contacted me after stumbling across this article, and who consider the effects of G-spot stimulation to be the highlight of their sexual pleasures, that they were totally healthy and actually ahead of the curve in terms of their sexual expression. We are all different, and there is no "right" way to obtain sexual pleasure. While the field of sexuality is rife with contradictions, we cannot deny clinical research any more than we can negate the testimonies of real women and their partners. Every woman has a G-spot (no matter how small or large) and therefore the possibility to reap the pleasure it can provide. Even if a woman has yet to unveil the powers of her own G-spot, its existence should not be ignored any more than it should become a source of anxiety. After all, as Beverly Whipple implied in her comments to the journalist from the BBC, what I call PGO (predominantly genitally oriented) sex is not conducive to the pleasures of the G-spot, which requires extended periods of arousal and direct contact for a positive response.

The G-spot becomes turgid and easy to locate when a woman is sexually aroused, with a finger, the sensitive tip of the penis, or any other object that may be used to penetrate the entryway to the vaginal canal. Being that most women consider the raised area that represents the G-spot to be the most sensitive area of their genitals, it should not be approached before the signals of heightened arousal have fully manifested. The enlargement of the G-spot, along with the dilation of the inner walls of the vagina and enhanced lubrication, is one of the most obvious signals of heightened arousal.

MASSAGE, STROKE, AND TICKLE

Some women's G-spots are larger or more defined than others, and, like the clitoris, once the G-spot has risen to the occasion, it is also surprisingly resilient and receptive to being stroked. If the woman in question is massaged with skillful intent and she is relaxed enough to abandon herself to its powers, the G-spot orgasm may manifest. Over extended periods of arousal, the paraurethral glands and ducts that comprise the female prostate become engorged with ejaculate fluid, and direct stimulation of the G-spot may provoke emission. When the ejaculation reflex is prompted, the fluid produced in the female prostate exits the body through the urethra, not through the vagina, in unmistakable jets and streams. The quantity of the fluid emitted can range from a few drops to much more, depending on the levels of arousal, awareness, and abandonment of the woman.

Since only six to eight percent of sexually mature females report that they ejaculate, we may assume that the female prostate and the related phenomenon of ejaculation have nothing to do with the procreative process at all. Women who enjoy G-spot stimulation consider it to be the catalyst for the most intense pleasures that they can experience. The prostate gland is explored in detail in relation to the pleasures of G-spot stimulation and female emission in the chapter "Navigating the Sacred River: Female Emissions."

Beyond the G-spot, there are other highly sensitive zones located within the vaginal canal that are capable of providing deeply pleasurable sensations. The most noted is the A-spot, or AFE zone (anterior fornix erogenous zone), discovered by the Malaysian sex researcher Dr. Chua Chee Ann in the early 1990s. The spongy composition of this highly sensitive area lies deep inside the anterior wall of the vaginal canal, near the cervix. Known to be more extensive yet less defined than the G-spot, the A-spot is capable of provoking comparably vivid orgasmic responses. Sensitizing the A-spot requires deep penetration with the penis or the fingers. It responds to a softer touch than the G-spot and stimulates increased lubrication.

Applying pressure to the female perineum either directly or indirectly, through vaginal or anal penetration, stimulates what is known as the perineal sponge—the termination of the dense portion of the clitoral system known as the vestibular bulbs.

In males, the Cowper's glands lie within the perineal wall. They emit the clear, slick, alkaline Cowper's fluid, commonly called pre-cum. Pre-cum neutralizes the acidic environment of the urinary canal caused by the trace presence of urine to guarantee the sperms' safe journey to the outside world. Some men emit Cowper's fluid long before they actually ejaculate. In others, pre-cum indicates heightened levels of arousal and imminent ejaculation. Note that because pre-cum may contain sperm, withdrawal is an ineffective method of birth control.

Stroking the male perineum permits indirect contact with the prostate gland and the vas deferens, the duct that moves sperm and male hormones, including testosterone, from the testicles through the male apparatus by peristalsis, or smooth muscle wall contractions. Once the sperm exit the testicles, they make a stopover in the seminal sacs, or vesicles, where seminal fluid is added to the vital mixture, which is then pushed along with the help of the vas deferens until it reaches the prostate gland. During this final pit stop, prostate fluid is added to the recipe, and the sperm are finally readied for their mission. At the moment of ejaculation, semen exits the prostate gland and moves toward the urethral opening. When it has completely filled the urethra, this applies pressure to the prostate gland, provoking the fluttering sensation that most men recognize as imminent, and usually unavoidable, ejaculation. This signals the beginning of the sperm's outward race. Learning to recognize these sensations and control the vas deferens before this occurs is crucial to the evolution of the Sexual Ceremony, when male partners are involved. We will examine this sexual skill in the chapter "Riding the Orgasmic Wave: Male Ejaculation Control."

During the Paradise Found Sexual Ceremony, the areas directly surrounding the sexual organs, male or female, are as important as the genitals themselves. The fine skin of the inner thighs is highly sensitive and capable of providing ecstatic sensations. For women, the pubic triangle, or the mons pubis, has soft, sensitive flesh that responds well to being massaged, stroked, and tickled. For men and women, the perineum, which creates a bridge between the genitals and the anus, responds well to deep strokes and decisive pressure.

Understanding your body and that of your lover's allows you to create a map that will guide you both on your journeys to heightened sexual satisfaction. In addition, to know your genitals better is to take responsibility for them and the pleasure they can provide. This is fundamental to your capacity to accept, enhance, and share the *joie du sexe* that lies ahead.

CHAPTER 2

———————o———————

COAXING THE SEXUAL VIBRATION:
ENHANCING THE ORGASM

Reaching late his flower,
Round her chamber hums—
Counts his nectars—
Enters—and is lost in Balms.

— Emily Dickinson, "Come Slowly—Eden"

THE ORGASM IS ONE of the greatest rewards of our sexual endeavor, and learning to enhance its impact will obviously benefit our sense of satisfaction. While orgasms are not the only highlight of the sexual ritual, for most they are the gauge of its positive outcome.

What we know about orgasms is that they are a discharge of neuromuscular tensions, and the contractions they send rippling through the pelvic floor muscles, vibrating the entirety of the genitals, provide us with a kind of intense pleasure that is hard to describe! While often associated with ejaculation (particularly in men), the orgasm reflex is actually a separate bodily function from the ejaculation reflex. If you find that hard to believe, hark back to the pleasures you procured through masturbation, long before you were sexually mature. These experiences are proof, especially for men, that orgasm and ejaculation are two very distinct, and separable, reflexes.

Like the functions of the body's vital organs, the functions of the orgasm are commanded by the autonomic nervous system and therefore operate beyond our conscious control. We cannot "climax" on command any more than we can keep from breathing or halt our heartbeat. We can, however, positively influence our vital organs' functioning through healthy practices such as exercise and good nutrition. Similarly, we can learn to experience more deeply gratifying, full-body orgasms by enhancing our sexual awareness, understanding, and skills. This includes recognizing and changing behavioral patterns that inhibit rather than enhance pleasure. Keep in mind, however, that because each orgasm has its own unrepeatable identity, trying to reach the same pleasure twice will likely diminish, if not inhibit altogether, an orgasm's impact.

The degree of desire and attraction between partners also influences the orgasmic wave. While occasional partners who are obliged to use barriers will not be able to indulge in a complete exchange of sexual energy, if they truly desire each other, they may still experience elevated levels of sexual satisfaction. The more intimate lovers are, the more likely they are to truly abandon themselves to each other, which is fundamental to experiencing heightened degrees of orgasmic pleasure. What deep trust can do for enhanced pleasure cannot be undervalued.

EROTIC MEDITATION

To build ever-greater levels of intimacy, consider your erotic playtime a form of meditation. Be present and truly venerate each other by focusing on what you are doing to your lover and what is being done to you. Lack of concentration is the primary reason for premature ejaculation in men and for what was once termed frigidity in women. No one wants to be in bed with a distracted, clumsy lover! Whether you are pleasing yourself or someone is pleasuring you, it is crucial to be in the moment.

The positive effects of your attention will be even more rewarding if you learn to visualize the sexual energy as it mounts within the system. The Indian surgeon Sushruta (circa 600 B.C.), in the *Sushruta Samhita*, described the vital essence as ". . . invisible currents of zigzag swirling patterns . . . like waves of sound, in an upward direction like flames of fire, and in a downward direction like rivulets of water."

Psycho-sensual visualization evolves from the interaction of the mind with the senses, and it has been practiced by every culture that considers sex sacred. The conscious visualization of the flow of sexual energy in association with deep, controlled breathing patterns has a radiating effect. During extended periods of arousal, lovers can learn to "pull" the energy generated in the genitals and "weave" it throughout the entire body.

You might also try visualizing the object of worship. An early Hindu text invited male lovers to "think of the sexual region of a woman as a sacrificial altar, her hairs as the sacrificial grass, her skin as the elixir dispenser, the two lips of her Yoni [female genitals] as the tongues of flame that rise up from the offering." Hindi women were invited to visualize the lingam (penis) as the living embodiment of the transcendental force—the god Shiva. Set your imagination free and allow your own psycho-sensual visualizations to manifest. Reinforcing the mind-body-spirit interrelation will enhance the orgasm's impact.

Become aware of how the orgasm reflex manifests in your body. The next time you are on the verge of an orgasm, observe what is happening. Are you in a state of physical tension rather than relaxation? Are your legs, buttocks, shoulders, back, and neck taut? Are you holding your breath? If so, you are on the verge of having a tension orgasm—a common, unconscious habit related to "fast sex." Muscular rigidity increases when we hold our breath, which does not allow the orgasmic wave to mount to its full potential. While tension may permit us to cum faster, it actually slows rather than facilitates the flow of blood to the genitals, resulting in genitally localized sensations that more closely resemble repressed sneezes than deep, rolling waves of full-body pleasure. While tension orgasms can come in handy if you have no time or energy for anything but a "quickie," they reveal only a fraction of our orgasmic pleasure capacity.

Learn to relax into your pleasure. Remind yourself to breathe into the sensations you are experiencing as your pleasure mounts, rather than holding your breath. Deep, full breaths send pure oxygenated blood throughout the entire body, including the genitals. So *breathe* with ecstatic purpose: let fresh oxygen relax the mind and purify and enliven the entire body. A calm mind is a more creative mind, which leads the body to become more receptive to pleasure. The disciplines of yoga and meditation incorporate breath awareness and control in the earliest stages of the practice. Their techniques can be utilized in the Paradise Found Sexual Ceremony to great effect. As many yogis say, "Where the mind goes, the body follows."

ORGASMS: THE SEXUAL DANCE

Both the male and female genitals are nestled in a congregation of blood vessels. During arousal, blood surges into the penis and the clitoral system, and as pleasure mounts and crests, endorphins, the body's "love drug," are injected into the bloodstream, transporting us higher into the sexual dimension. Endorphins increase our tolerance to pain while chemically reinforcing our perception of pleasure. Over the course of a lengthy sexual ritual, they will also evoke a divine glow. Take a look at yourself in a mirror after you have flown on the wings of ecstasy, and you will see for yourself . . . there is simply no greater beauty enhancer than deeply gratifying sex.

Many people presume that men's and women's orgasms are exactly alike, but there are several crucial differences. For one, the mounting of sexual tension that leads to climax in women may take longer than it does in their male counterparts; however, the time shortens radically when women are masturbating alone and concentrating exclusively on their own pleasure. Because of this presumption of similarity, women who can't adapt to the limitations of sexual urgency during partner sex and arrive at the finish line with a single orgasm of their own were considered frigid. Today, however, we know that the inability to experience orgasm during partner sex is linked to a question of timing. "Fast sex" does not allow a woman, any more than it permits a man, to explore her multifaceted pleasure capacity or savor truly deep levels of sexual satisfaction.

Another crucial difference between male and female orgasms is that when men ejaculate during orgasm, it is usually a signal of the end of the sexual encounter. In order to attain another erection and achieve orgasm again, men are obliged to wait and often rest. The time it takes to recuperate from ejaculation depends upon the man's age, health, and level of desire. The female orgasm, on the other hand, even if it is associated with ejaculation, does not interrupt the mounting of the woman's sexual pleasures nor necessarily mark the end of the sexual encounter. While a woman may become hypersensitive after achieving orgasm (and perhaps need a brief pause from direct contact with her clitoris), lengthy phases of recuperation are not required in order for her to experience consecutive climaxes. On the contrary, if her lover is generous and skilled in the art of loving, a woman's first climax marks only the beginning of the sexual dance, and she may climax repeatedly, such as throughout the duration of the Paradise Found Sexual Ceremony.

Since the 1980s, a great deal of attention has been dedicated to understanding the phenomenon of multiple orgasms in women.

Clinical research reveals that all women are potentially multi-orgasmic, and their capacity to experience manifold waves of pleasure is determined primarily by their desire to do so! The phenomenon can be linked to an anatomical difference between the male and female genitals.

The penis contains a venous plexus, a concentrated congregation of blood vessels. During arousal, blood rushes into the penis via this venous plexus and remains trapped in the erectile tissues by the contraction of the pelvic muscles, once the organ has assumed its fully erect state. During orgasm, the spinal medulla induces a sudden relaxation of the muscular tension, and the flow of blood into the genitals via the venous plexus is reversed, marking the end of the erection.

Within the female genitals, the formation of the venous plexus is not nearly as concentrated, so the blood flow to and from the genitals is facilitated. This difference in the formation of the venous plexus may be the principal biological explanation for multiple orgasms. Even though the blood engorges the female genitals during arousal in a similar fashion to the male's, after the point of female orgasm, once the wave of pleasure has crested and subsided, more orgasms may ensue as long as both partners are ready to provide and receive the attention required to encourage blood to surge back into the genitals. The desire of a woman's partner to continue to provide orgasmic pleasures is as important as her desire to revel in such delights. Women should feel free to "help" their partners generate the powers of multiple orgasms by masturbating themselves, even to orgasm, during the shared pleasures of the Sexual Ceremony. Both partners are guaranteed to benefit from the results!

Women who experience multiple orgasms report increasing levels of intensity with each consecutive climax, rather than the diminishing of intensity acknowledged by men who orgasm and ejaculate more than once during the same encounter. This gradual mounting of pleasure is in part linked to an increase in the production of endorphins. Women who learn to explore their multiorgasmic capacity are likely to find that the release of sexual tension that a single orgasm provides leaves them feeling more eager than fulfilled. Men who learn to delay the ejaculation reflex and benefit from the pleasures of the internal orgasm will have a similar experience.

Women who have not yet explored their innate multiorgasmic capacity could be said to have "masculinized" their orgasms in order to correspond physically to male partners who themselves have probably not yet explored the benefits of male ejaculation delay. It is important that women not be expected to climax in time with the male and with the same urgency. It is by means of the male's ejaculation control that his partner is permitted to explore his or her orgasmic capacity to the greatest extent. These benefits and techniques are further described in the chapter "Riding the Orgasmic Wave: Male Ejaculation Control."

PATHS TO THE FEMALE ORGASM

In 1905, after analyzing the differences between female orgasms in association with vaginal penetration and those born from purely clitoral contact, the psychoanalyst Sigmund Freud stated that women who did not experience orgasms from penetration were sexually immature. Today it is commonly understood that the majority of women do not actually experience orgasm through penetration alone, but through direct or indirect clitoral stimulation and/or contact with the G-spot or the A-spot during the act of penetration.

In fact, sexually experienced women report having four different kinds of orgasms: from the clitoris, the G-spot, the U-spot, and from the A-spot, or the anterior fornix erogenous (AFE) zone. There are also women—and men—who report having orgasms without any genital contact at all, but simply via mental fantasy; during the practice of Kegel exercises; or through the stimulation of nipples, ears, neck, buttocks, or the feet. Both men and women are even capable of having orgasms during sleep—the body is, in fact, an incredible organism!

The clitoris is, however, the most common source of the female orgasm. Primarily fueled by the pudendal nerve, the pleasures that the clitoris provides are genitally localized. Orgasms that are linked to the A-spot and the G-spot provoke deeper sensations, as well as the potential for more emotional responses—even catharsis. This is due to the fact that both these spots are connected to the emotional centers of the brain by the powerful pelvic splanchnic nerve. Because expressing emotions opens the heart, these types of orgasms are known to increase the sense of intimacy between partners.

RITUAL MASTURBATION

Self-knowledge and awareness facilitate sexual communication, which increases the likelihood that your partner will be able to acknowledge and provide you with what pleases you most. When we are familiar and comfortable with our genitals, it is easier to invite our lovers to assist and share in the pleasures they provide, without inhibition.

We tend to masturbate in a hurry as a means of discharging sexual tension. Approaching masturbation as a ritual entails setting more time aside for pleasuring yourself—to explore the body and experience the effects of new sensations before sharing them with a lover. Ritual masturbation can be used to map the body's sensory range of pleasure. By becoming aware of your own responses to different forms of stimulation, and even observing yourself in a mirror, you will better understand your own desires (see plate I, page 65). Nothing is sexier than a lover who knows what she or he needs.

Many people associate masturbation with solitude and moments when sex with a partner is not possible. This has perpetuated one of the greatest myths surrounding masturbation: that we should stop pleasuring ourselves once we are in a happy relationship. Those who continue to masturbate on their own despite being in a relationship are often wrongly considered to be sexually unsatisfied. In reality, masturbation increases readiness in women, and as long as it is not practiced merely as a means to orgasm in association with ejaculation by men, it is a great way to increase desire for a partner's loving attention. Masturbation has the advantage of keeping the genitals toned and ready for action. Like any other muscle in the body, the pelvic-floor muscles that surround and support the sexual apparatus are healthier when they are regularly called into action. Masturbating together or inviting your lover to watch you masturbate during partner sex is great fun and also demystifies the masturbation taboo. It can teach partners about each other's response to genital stimulation.

If you are not in a relationship or are between partners, practicing the ritual of self-loving on a regular basis will help to avoid the negative effects of sexual frustration as well as the possibility that the libido may go lax through erotic complacency. Masturbation will keep the body primed until someone with whom to celebrate the shared joys of the sexual ritual comes along. It also has the power to reverse the subliminal effects of culturally induced sexual taboos and repression. In addition, masturbation has the power to revive lazy libidos, to renew waning desire between established couples, and enhance the orgasmic response.

THE ELECTRIFYING PLEASURES OF VIBRATORS

Many women hail vibrators as being the implement that revealed their innate capacity to orgasm. Like many sex therapists, I frequently prescribe them to anorgasmic women. These days, the market for these pulsating prosthetics is booming, and vibrators have never been more accessible—or acceptable! However, vibrators tend to make clitoral orgasms the primary, if not exclusive, motivator toward stimulation. Women, take your time when using a vibrator—explore the entirety of the vulva and the vagina with your fingers as well as with the vibrator, and don't forget that the clitoral system, which radiates inward from the clitoris, is not limited to the "tender button" alone.

While men are not the primary target for vibrator sales, there is no reason why they should not partake in the electrifying pleasures that these tools can provide. A vibrator can be used to enhance the sensations of manual stimulation—men, just place it in the palm of your hand and proceed! Used for extraordinary anal or genital stimulation, vibrators are guaranteed to incite new and intensely different sensations during male masturbation. I encourage men to experiment with vibrators that are designed specifically for prostate stimulation, which usually have a smaller diameter (for easy insertion) and a slight curve to their form. Be prepared to enjoy, as these little tools can oscillate a man toward unprecedented states of ecstasy! Anal penetration is explored in greater detail in the chapter "The Anthems of Anal Sex: From Hygiene to Heavenly Pleasures."

Vibrators can be used to massage any part of the body—the inner thighs, the nipples, the back, the lips, the feet, and the neck—and are often marketed as massage tools in American stores in order to avoid sales restrictions in states where sex-related objects are still considered illegal. But rest assured, if it is phallic in shape, it is also intended to provide more intimate massages and relieve tension that is not necessarily stress related. (This explains the comical notice that these implements often sport, which reads: "This device should not be used over swollen or inflamed areas or skin eruptions. In the case of unexplained calf pain, consult physician." Obviously, if you have inflamed genitals, or their delicate skin presents open wounds, the last thing that you want to do is break out the vibes!)

Because vibrators tend to pulsate, rattle, and rock themselves to their own demise, it is advisable to invest in a couple of medium-priced ones with power and ranges that suit your taste and to replace them when necessary. If you wish to make a more serious investment, choose electrically operated or rechargeable vibrators. They will last longer and are more ecologically friendly, and they also tend to be slightly less noisy. While modern vibrators have near-silent functions and a wider range of variations than ever before, their hum is anything but erotic. Covering them with a blanket or towel will help muffle their rattle to a low purr.

Whether using vibrators during solo masturbation or to enhance the shared joys of the Paradise Found Sexual Ceremony, remember to allow the sexual tension to mount gradually, which will increase the orgasmic impact for both genders.

A WOMAN'S RIGHT TO CUM

In spite of the fact that the sole function of the clitoris is to provide the pleasures of orgasm, and that women are no longer "punished" as they used to be for accepting this pleasure, many women (and men) are still under the debilitating effects of societal taboos and have yet to embrace woman's innate capacity to cum. During sessions with anorgasmic women, I invariably find myself giving them "permission" to embrace their orgasms; I firmly believe that while achieving an orgasm should not be viewed as an obligation, there is absolutely no reason why women should not be reveling in the unique pleasures that orgasms provide.

If you are a woman who has yet to experience orgasm, do not pressure yourself to do so, but rather make the commitment to dedicate more time to the discovery of your innate orgasmic capacity. Practiced in a ritual context, and on regular basis, solo masturbation is the best means to discover your orgasmic response. If you continue to suffer from anorgasmia, do not pressure yourself—put expectations aside. Take the time you need to know yourself more intimately, and enhance your sexual relationship with yourself—sooner or later you will awaken your orgasmic response and revel in every pleasure it proffers.

The greatest inhibitor of the female orgasm is the simulated orgasm. Faking an orgasm during partner sex may stem from fear of letting go, from a lack of self-esteem, or simply from a desire to get "it" over with. Simulating your orgasms will inevitably lead to conflict both with yourself and your partner or partners. Women who fake their orgasms may be victims of guilt and shame, and beneath these negative emotions lurks the pleasure taboo. The simulated orgasm may even inhibit a woman from discovering her real orgasm. If you resort to feigning your pleasure in the belief that you must avoid offending your partner, stop now! Otherwise, your partner will continue to do exactly what he or she thinks is making you happy—while you will only make yourself more dissatisfied and frustrated.

As with anorgasmia, masturbation is this condition's most efficient and effective form of sexual self-help. Women, if you seek your orgasm with the aid of a vibrator, try wrapping it in a silk scarf or using it over your panties or the sheets rather than placing it directly on the genitals. This will help to avoid the orgasm-inhibiting effects of sensory overload over extended periods of stimulation. Another hint: use lower speeds, or alternate between higher and lower speeds. Over time, using excessive speeds could have a numbing effect.

THE RACE TO EJACULATE

Though "anorgasmia" and "frigidity" are terms used frequently in reference to women, men also suffer from not fully accepting or enjoying their orgasms to maximum capacity, with premature ejaculation being the primary symptom of a man's difficulty. A man who desires and cares for his partner, male or female, will enjoy taking the time to pleasure him or her. Since a woman's orgasm can require more time to manifest, a man's refusal to delay his emission may be an unconscious means of punishing her. While premature ejaculation fulfills, however superficially, his own immediate needs, it completely ignores the importance of the needs of his partner. There are men who genuinely suffer from physically based premature ejaculation, but 80 percent of male sexual performance problems are related to psychological dynamics rather than medical issues. They can, thus, be resolved when admitted to and confronted, preferably with the support of his partner and, when necessary, with the help of a sex therapist.

If you are a healthy man suffering from premature ejaculation or lack of pleasure even in association with orgasm, take the time to practice the masturbation ritual regularly. The majority of men still approach masturbation with a sense of urgency. Rather than racing to ejaculate, men should explore the advantages of slowing things down and strive to master the skill of ejaculation control during the masturbation ritual. Approaching masturbation in this way is crucial to reversing the negative effects of fast sex, both upon your own sexuality as well as that of your partner's. It is also an effective means to get in touch with your body and enhance your awareness, skill, and orgasms.

BETTER ORGASMS FOR BETTER HEALTH

Pleasure is the "glue" in long-term relationships, and the greater the pleasure, the happier the couple. The beneficial effects of a mutually satisfying sex life on the harmony and stability of a couple are undeniable. Learning to enhance the impact of the orgasm reflex will reinforce the pleasure bond by heightening your overall sense of satisfaction—and provide some unexpected benefits beyond the boudoir, as well. Clinical research reveals that orgasms reduce stress and, therefore, the risk of heart attacks. They alleviate headaches, migraines, and overall aches and pains, including those related to menstruation. By increasing the circulation of fresh, oxygenated blood into the genitals, orgasms reduce the risk of endometriosis as well as cervical and urinary tract infections in women. By eliminating carcinogenic toxins from the body, orgasms also reduce the risk of both prostate and uterine cancer. Orgasms have the advantage of improving the overall health of the skin, balancing the brain's chemistry, and boosting the immune system. They also strengthen the pelvic floor muscles crucial to enhanced satisfaction. The positive effects of great orgasms upon our health and well-being are as important as the effects of our general health and well-being are upon our sense of sexual satisfaction. Great orgasms cannot exist without good health, and vice versa, so take good care of yourself in every way!

A WORD ON PORN: DEBUNKING THE MYTHS

If a thing is worth doing, it is worth doing slowly . . . very slowly.

— Gypsy Rose Lee

PORNOGRAPHY HELPED to liberate the female orgasm in the 1970s by portraying women taking their pleasure on-screen. It also helped to perpetuate the concept of sex for sex's sake. But over time, it has also established itself as the world's worst sex-education teacher. With all due respect for the industry and the men and women who keep the XXX-rated cameras rolling, let's analyze some of the pleasure-inhibiting myths that pornography commonly glorifies. Don't be surprised if you discover that you have a bit of unlearning to do!

MYTH #1: FAST EQUALS SKILLFUL

The pornographic film industry's glorification of the emission of semen as the ultimate pleasure can be held partly responsible for the fact that ejaculation remains, for most, the principal goal of sex. Lovers, both male and female, have wrongly learned to associate sexual skill with the ability to bring a male partner to ejaculate in record-breaking time.

In reality, the emission of semen is not a sure sign that a male partner has been pleased; men can ejaculate without benefiting at all from the pleasures of an orgasm. Associating rapid ejaculation with sexual skill eventually causes frustration—both in the (seemingly) satisfied male in question and his partner, whether male or female.

MYTH #2: REPEATED EMISSION EQUALS SEXUAL PROWESS

Why is it that nothing sells XXX-rated flicks, homosexual or heterosexual, better than urgent, repeated, abundant emissions of semen? The reason is that the sex industry is directed predominantly by and for men. Viewers want to see cum (and lots of it) because those little spermatozoa, not ejaculation control, are the ultimate symbols of male virility.

While there are exceptions to every rule, a single emission normally amounts to an average of one or two teaspoons of the vital fluid. The impressive "cum shots" glorified by the porn industry have more to do with editing and stunts than reality. But for whatever reason, fact or fiction, abundant ejaculation scenes are what viewers have been taught to expect and enjoy.

MYTH #3: THE EVER-READY ROCK-HARD PHALLUS

I discovered, during my consultations with men who suffer from performance anxiety, that many of them were avid "pornivores." Most of these men had convinced themselves that their erectile performance, like their emissions, was "unworthy" in comparison to those of their pornographic role models. But a penis that is commanded by the laws of attraction and desire should not be compared to the often chemically enhanced erection of a pornographic role model—a "stud" who may work five days per week (and more, if required) and ejaculate up to four times a day!

Consider that the footage for an average 120-minutes porn flick is normally filmed over the course of 1 to 6 long days. Everyone on the playbill is expected to rise and perform until the film is complete, a feat that would be impossible for most adult males to achieve naturally. Porn stars work hard, in every sense of the word! In order to keep the cameras rolling with low budgets and restricted time limits, male porn stars, no matter how skilled they may be, cannot rely on Mother Nature alone. Erection enhancers permit male performers to exceed the limits of nature; in fact, if Viagra and its like had not been invented, pornography would still be a niche market, not the booming industry it is today.

Also keep in mind that what comes across as one long, libidinous act is generally the result of several scenes that are cut and spliced together to create a pornographic whole. Master shots are edited with close-ups and cum shots. Fake semen is often used to enhance the visual impact of the scene: a few strategic squirts of creamy hair conditioner or milky lubricating gel will make an average cum scene camera worthy! If a performer has taken an erection enhancer yet is unable to emit in a timely fashion, he might slip on a condom, the tip of which is pierced after it has been filled with mock semen. A few decisive strokes of a skilled hand . . . and voilà, the desired visuals!

MYTH #4: THE BIGGER THE BETTER

Another myth sustained by pornography is that bigger penises are better when it comes to orgasmic potential, which has no basis in reality. In a porn film, the penis is the star of the show and, as such, must be visible at all times even during scenes that involve lots of body contact, including penetration; the use of monumental close-ups as well as highly creative camera angles thus glorify massive members.

The issue of size is a great source of performance anxiety, which is, in turn, a primary orgasm inhibitor, and not only for the man in question but also for his partner. In the scheme of orgasmic sex, *big* is simply not synonymous with *skillful*. Similarly, the size of the penis does not determine male sexual superiority any more than it determines a man's capacity to provide or receive pleasure.

Men, I urge you to put your anatomical concerns aside! Learn to extend playtime and to love and accept your genitals, whatever their size or shape, and you will be less likely to suffer the negative effects of performance anxiety. Research has proven that most men who feel inadequate are actually perfectly within the average range.

Consider this: our Greco-Roman forefathers appreciated the proportions of smaller penises over larger, which they considered *vulgaris*! No matter where you happen to find yourself on the measuring stick, fuel your imagination and experiment with creative ways to provide pleasure beyond penetration alone. Men who accept their natural disposition, whatever it may be, and learn to express themselves skillfully without shame or inhibition are bound not only to have (and provide) better orgasms but to enjoy healthier, happier sexual relations, too.

Seek and you shall find the partner that corresponds to your size and shape. The ancient Indian sex guides *Kama Sutra* and *Ananga Ranga* both expound on the importance of compatibility. "When the proportions of both lovers are alike and equal, then satisfaction is easy to achieve," proclaims the *Ananga Ranga*, which uses six different animals to illustrate the ideal sexual connection between differing dimensions of the lingam, or the penis, and depths of the yoni, or the vagina:

· Small: hare for man, deer for woman
· Medium: bull for man, mare for woman
· Large: horse for man, elephant for woman

Unequal unions—for example, between a hare and an elephant—are likely to decrease the levels of pleasure and comfort that lovers can expect to experience.

MYTH #5: SAFE IS NOT SEXY

A no-condom policy exists in the porn industry, because statistics reveal that the use of condoms in a porn film radically reduces its commercial success. Because barriers such as condoms are rarely used, porn stars must test for HIV and other STDs on a more-than-regular basis; even this, sadly, does not always prevent the actors from contracting a disease, any more than it does in the real world. So use the visuals of pornography to fuel your fantasies, not as an example to follow. If you are not in an established and safe fluid-exchange agreement, condoms and regular blood tests should be considered an obligation.

Another risky practice that is commonly represented in heterosexual and female-to-female pornography is anal-to-vaginal penetration. Whether it is performed with a finger, a penis, or any other object of desire, careless anal-to-vaginal contact is likely to lead to serious vaginal infections, so avoid making this discomforting mistake at all costs.

MYTH #6: WOMAN AS EVER-READY PROVIDER

Pornographers also tend to ignore the importance of foreplay as well as the relevance of sentiment in relation to sexual satisfaction. These values, so vital to deep sexual satisfaction, cannot be communicated without a storyline, and unlike some of the porn that was created in the 1970s, contemporary porn rarely has a story to tell—with the exception of the subliminal "plot" that the female partner is at her best as a submissive and ever-ready provider of sex to the dominant or omnipotent male partner. A woman who aspires to "make love like a porn star" may, without realizing it, be reinforcing such an archaic role model. By begging a lover to give it to her *"Fast! And hard! In my face! And now!"* and opting to forget the relevance of her own pleasure, she becomes an accomplice in phallocentrism.

A surprising number of women compensate for their inability to accept the gift of sexual pleasure by concentrating solely on giving pleasure. Their partners are therefore subject to a similar one-sided consequence—they more often receive than provide. Great sex is an exchange; it requires that we learn to enjoy being pleased as much as our lovers expect us to enjoy pleasuring them. By re-evaluating the importance of our own pleasure, as well as providing for that of our lovers, we can make a contribution toward mutually enhanced sexual satisfaction. Partner sex is proactive. Skilled lovers, no matter their sexual orientation, should enjoy taking each other to Paradise!

MYTH #7: THE HYSTERICAL ARCH

Another anti-orgasmic lesson disseminated by pornography and most readily exemplified and imitated by women is represented by what sexologist Wilhelm Reich defined as the *hysterical arc de cercle*, or the hysterical arch (see plate IV, page 68). This position is commonly assumed by a woman when she is lying on her back: she presses her buttocks firmly downward while arching her lower back, which in turn causes the pelvis to rock both forward and down. When a woman is thus posed to pornographic perfection, her head is thrown savagely back, which causes the lips to part, resulting in the ultimate symbol of female readiness and seduction.

There is nothing wrong with striking this pose for the sake of aesthetics, but it is important to know that, for a woman, indulging in the hysterical arch is guaranteed to diminish, if not completely inhibit, the orgasmic impact, as pressing the genitals downward in this manner blocks the blood flow into the entire pelvic area. (Note that men who assume this position are subject to similar orgasm-inhibiting physiological responses, which they can use to a positive end to delay their orgasm. The chapter "Riding the Orgasmic Wave: Male Ejaculation Control" details the advantages of what I term the "control arch" when it is used by men.)

For women, inverting the hysterical arch will facilitate and heighten the pleasures inherent to orgasm. Simply "inverse" the pose (see plate IV, page 68): press your lower back against the surface on which you are resting, and roll your hips up rather than down. Let your head fall forward toward your sternum, so that your upper body will assume a U shape rather than a backward arch. Though the position may not make you look like a porn star, it will direct the flow of blood toward the center of the body and deeply enhance the depth, breadth, and intensity of every orgasm.

MYTH #8: SEX IS FOR THE YOUTHFUL

Our society's association of sexual pleasure with youth is reinforced by the pornography industry. There is, admittedly, no "bull market" for bodies that are older or out of shape. But there are no age limits for ecstasy! Sexual satisfaction should be considered a fundamental part of our overall well-being, indifferent to our age; orgasms should accompany us throughout our adult lives. (And if one could choose, wouldn't an earth-shattering orgasm be the ideal way to go?)

Unfortunately, many mature women still believe that after a certain age, they should not (and will not) be interested in sexual pleasure. While the maturing woman's body does undergo a gradual reduction of estrogen, the female sex hormone, the mighty myth of "no sex after fifty" is another anti-pleasure dogma whose influence we ought to shed. After fifty, our sex lives do not cease to exist; they simply evolve.

A mature woman's orgasmic capacity has nothing to do with her procreative function; on the contrary, by the time women reach the age of fifty they may have knowledge enough to be less inhibited and more capable of reaching orgasmic heights. In fact, in Japan, a geisha's value was increased with the arrival of her menopause.

Like women, mature men experience a gradual drop in hormone production, including testosterone, the male sex hormone. The phenomenon is known as andropause, or "male menopause." This hormonal decrease may lead to a gradual decline in the sexual impulse and what men describe as "slowing down." Andropause may also be accompanied by occasional bouts of impotence and moodiness. But as long as a man has not become clinically impotent, this seemingly unfortunate condition has some hidden benefits.

Andropause allows men to extend sexual playtime and enables them to step back from phallocentric goals to explore the body as a sexual whole. Mature men tend to have good ejaculation control, so while a mature man may require more coaxing and manipulation to encourage the penis to full erection, this fact of nature does not signify that his pleasure is any less intense than in the past. Keep in mind that a man does not have to have an erection, nor achieve ejaculation, in order to experience pleasure.

In fact, the most detrimental thing that a man can do to his erection, and thus to his orgasm, is to place himself under psychological pressure to "perform." While a man's erection may not rise to attention as automatically it did in his youth, the bright side of getting older is that a youthful, energetic sexual performance will be replaced with the advanced skills a man has acquired by the time he has reached maturity. Men, accept the physical changes that occur in the genitals as an organic part of the maturation process, and realize that you are at a height of sexual capacity—

you are able both to give and receive extended sexual pleasures with greater ease.

So dismantle and replace those die-hard myths and misconceptions that surround the pleasures of orgasm with sexual commonsense. Permit yourself greater pleasure, no matter your age or sexual orientation. If you like to observe sexual scenes on film, think about recording your own "real sex" movies. But don't let pornographic ideals interfere with your satisfaction—whether the camera is rolling or not.

This Cannot Be Ignored!
Statistics reveal that ninety percent of children between the ages of eight and sixteen have viewed pornography online, often involuntarily stumbling across hard-core material while doing homework, and eighty percent of fifteen- to seventeen-year-olds have had multiple hard-core exposures—these statistics cannot be ignored. When information regarding not only the dangers of sex but also the importance of a healthy sexuality is given to adolescents in schools, a new era of sexual enlightenment will commence. I am convinced that such an education would bestow inestimable benefits upon society. It is also the only way to counteract the negative effects that pornography is wreaking on the sexual development of children today.

CHAPTER 3

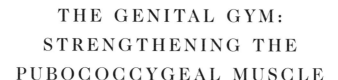

THE GENITAL GYM: STRENGTHENING THE PUBOCOCCYGEAL MUSCLE

Once again limb-loosening Eros shakes me, a helpless crawling thing, sweet-bitter.

— Sappho

FRESH, OXYGENATED BLOOD, delivered throughout the body by regular exercise, is critical to the health of every organ and muscle. The muscles that sustain the position of the genitals likewise suffer from lack of exercise. Suspended like a sling between the pubic bone and tailbone is the pubococcygeal muscle, a.k.a. the PC muscle (see plates II and III, pages 66 and 67). The openings of the urethra, the anus, and, in women, the vagina pass through this muscle. In both sexes, the perineum is the area where the PC muscle lies closest to the surface. While women who have given birth are more likely to be familiar with techniques that strengthen the PC muscle, such as Kegel exercises, PC muscle tonicity is pertinent to all women's genital health and pleasure, as well as men's, as there is a direct connection between the vigor of one's genital muscles and the orgasmic impact.

There is no single sport that directly reinforces the PC muscle better than sex itself, but those who practice yoga or Pilates are likely to have developed PC muscle awareness and control through the practice of Mula Bandha, which calls into action the sphincter muscles, the vaginal muscles, and, in certain moments, the entirety of the PC muscle. In yogic vocabulary, *bhanda* signifies unification, blocking, or contraction, and it almost always refers to gestures or positions that serve to control the muscles that surround the orifices of the body. Bhanda also influences the circulation of blood, the nervous system, and the endocrine glands.

Like yoga, Kegel exercises improve and maintain the health of the PC muscle. These exercises were developed and prescribed by Dr. Arnold Kegel in 1948 as a postpartum cure for childbirth-related incontinence and for the restoration of vaginal muscle strength. His female patients reported that the exercises not only strengthened the PC muscle, resolving any urinary incontinence, but also made the vagina tighter and enhanced orgasmic pleasure. Dr. Kegel concluded that increasing PC muscle strength amplifies the transmission of sensations to nerve endings in the genitals, leading to the intensification of the orgasm.

The Taoist and Tantric disciplines of erotic loving place great emphasis on PC tone and health, because genital muscle control is central to the techniques of ejaculation delay in men and to the orgasm and the ejaculation reflexes in women. Practitioners use the PC muscle to coax the sexual vibration to radiate from its source throughout the entire body. Taoists call PC-related exercises "sexual kung fu"; I call the exercises that enhance PC muscle strength and develop heightened genital awareness in both men and women the "PC muscle flex."

FOR POWERFUL PLEASURES: THE PC MUSCLE FLEX

First, locate your PC muscle and test its strength; the easiest way is during urination. Women should sit wide-legged on the toilet; men may either stand before the toilet or sit down on it, and they, too, should keep their legs spread wide.

As you urinate, try to stop and restart the flow, repeatedly, until your bladder is empty, noting as you do the corresponding tightening and relaxing of the PC muscle. If you are able to perform this test with ease, your PC muscles are probably in fairly good shape. However, if you have difficulty controlling the flow of urine, you should make the following exercises a priority in your daily health routine.

Initiate the genital gym by focusing your full attention on the genital area and using your inhalations and exhalations as a metronome to create a rhythm. Begin on an inhalation and simultaneously tighten the PC muscle in its entirety, from the tailbone to the pubic bone. You will feel the muscle twitch as it draws the genitals upward and inward.

Then, on the exhalation, gradually push the muscle downward and then relax the muscle completely. Repeat the exercise, in a slow rhythm (a five-second-long breath, for example), by contracting the PC muscle with each inhalation and then gently pushing it downward and relaxing it with each exhalation. As freshly oxygenated blood rushes to this muscle, you will experience a warm, tingling sensation, just as with any other repetitive exercise. It not only feels good, but it is good for you!

Once you become familiar with the exercise and begin to build PC muscle strength, start to increase the duration of your inhalations and exhalations and/or alternate the rhythm of the PC muscle flex. For example, do quick sets of five to twenty-five consecutive contractions on each inhalation, and then relax the muscle as you exhale to the count of five, ten, or more.

Another variation is an inversion of the rhythm: tense the muscle upon inhalation, and upon exhalation maintain the tension for a count of ten. Upon the next inhalation, on a count of five, gently push the muscle downward and then relax. While there is no right number of contractions to execute, gradually adding to the duration of your workout will further reinforce the PC muscle's tone. Alternating between faster and slower sets of muscle contractions creates a deeper PC muscle workout, which in turn leads to greater control. To assess your progress, practice the strength test during urination.

You can practice the genital gym with absolute discretion almost anywhere, while seated or standing, at any moment of the day! For example, if you are obliged to wait your turn in line at the bank or post office, a round of the genital gym will pass the time more pleasantly. Best of all, no one will notice your efforts, but both you and your lover are guaranteed to enjoy the results.

You will soon notice that muscular strength isn't the only benefit to practicing the PC muscle flex; this exercise makes for a genital meditation that not only reinforces that muscle, enhancing orgasmic pleasures, but also greatly heightens concentration and induces a powerful sense of clarity and well-being.

GRIP, SUCK, HUG: ENJOYING THE BENEFITS

Once you have greater PC muscle control, the genital gym may be enjoyed during solo masturbation and incorporated into the Sexual Ceremony to transcendent effect.

First, you need a "grip point" upon which to flex the muscle. Penetrating the vagina or anus with a finger or fingers, or with the penis or any phallus-shaped accessory will do. An especially effective alternative for the anus is an implement designed specifically for anal pleasure, like a stimulator for the male P-spot (the prostate) or anal beads or Ben Wa balls. Using a grip point will enhance the sensational effects of the exercises and invite the sexual vibration to expand even farther.

Contract the vaginal or anal muscles surrounding the implement of choice; then, while tightening the PC muscle, try to pull the object gently from the orifice. Create resistance by gripping the object harder—try to prevent it from leaving the body. This forces the PC muscles to work more intensely and provides a more strenuous (and ecstatically effective) workout.

You can train yourself to "suck" the object of penetration into your vagina or anus during the inward thrust and then embrace the penetrator as it withdraws in a warm, soft "hug" by gently pushing your PC muscle down and relaxing. Learning to pull in and push out in this manner provides ecstatic sensations and is critical to a woman's ability to control the genital muscles during female ejaculation. It is equally effective in the context of male ejaculation control.

GOOD VIBRATIONS: BEN WA BALLS

Ben Wa balls, also known as geisha balls because of their association with traditional Japanese erotica, may be used as vaginal "grips" to enhance the effects of the genital gym. Normally worn in pairs (though the single egg-shaped version works equally well), these slick, smooth spherical objects may also be hollow and contain another sphere within that provides extra vibrations. Like most sexual accessories, Ben Wa balls are considered to be "gadgets" and so are rarely sold with instructions for their correct and safe use—what follows can serve as a guide, but there is no substitute for common sense!

Historically made of ivory or even metals containing lead, Ben Wa balls today are most often composed of plastic or unidentified metals whose toxicity levels are under-evaluated or unknown. So unless you are sure that the Ben Wa balls' materials will not provoke negative side effects, use a barrier before inserting them into your body. Best would be to choose Ben Wa balls made of hygienic, body-safe materials such as surgical stainless steel or precious metals such as sterling silver or 18-karat gold. I do not recommend using objects that are plated in silver or gold; surface scratches will expose base metals like nickel and brass, which are not body safe.

Some Ben Wa balls are strung on a synthetic cord; these models may also be inserted into the anus, as long as a portion of the cord remains outside the body. Ben Wa balls that do not have cords are designed for vaginal use only—never insert Ben Wa balls that do not have a retrieval cord into the anus! (For that matter, do not insert *any* object into the anus unless it has a cord, a flared end, or is long enough to grasp, otherwise it is likely you will need to see a doctor to have it removed.) Note that the cord for Ben Wa balls is difficult to thoroughly sterilize. Therefore Ben Wa balls that have been used in the rectum must be reserved for that purpose alone.

Smaller, cordless Ben Wa balls made of acrylic or other hard plastics (a material that is generally more body safe than soft plastics) or hygienic metals may be worn in the vagina even during penetration. Their slick, round surfaces will provide a sense of full-ness, offering extra-pleasurable sensations for both partners. Choose smaller Ben Wa balls for shared pleasures and larger Ben Wa balls for exercising the PC muscles. It is important to note that pregnant women should not use Ben Wa balls during penetration, though they are highly recommended before and after childbirth to heighten vaginal awareness, restore PC muscle strength, and thereby cure postpartum urinary incontinence.

Many women may refrain from experimenting with Ben Wa balls, especially models that aren't strung on cords, from the commonly held and mistaken fear that the balls might get stuck in the vaginal canal or even disappear inside the uterus. Unless a woman is in the very last phases of pregnancy, the opening in the cervix that leads to the uterus is no larger than a pinhole, so it is impossible that a pair of Ben Wa balls, or any other sexual device, could be lost inside the body.

I am often asked, "How does one remove cordless Ben Wa balls from the vagina?" It is as simple as squatting and inserting a finger into the vagina to coax them down and out. If they have been used during intercourse, they might have gotten pushed deep into the vaginal canal—but don't panic! Women, if you cannot retrieve them immediately with ease, put on a pair of panties, take a walk, and they will begin to shift and descend. Do not remove metal Ben Wa balls over tile floors or other hard surfaces. Should they hit the floor, their spherical forms may be scratched or dented, providing havens for germs.

Some women like to wear Ben Wa balls beyond the boudoir for the continuous vibrations they can provide in the vagina and to build genital awareness. Of course, this will spark up daily tasks, but make sure you don't lose your train of thought while running an errand!

MOVE TO THE GROOVE: THE PELVIC SWING

Pelvic rigidity is a common condition that negatively affects one's posture by slowing the free flow of energy along the spinal cord and inhibiting the circulation of fresh, oxygenated blood throughout the entire body. The effect that pelvic rigidity has upon our capacity to experience sexual satisfaction should not be underestimated.

The source of much pelvic rigidity is the gender conditioning to which most of us were subject, from the earliest stages of our childhood. Little boys are told to control the sway of their hips, as that gesture is deemed inappropriately feminine (and therefore associated with homosexuality). Little girls are told not to swing their hips because it is considered "naughty." In either case, pelvic sways are viewed as a blatant indication of sexual knowledge and so deemed inappropriate for young children.

By the time most of us reach adulthood, we have learned to

constrain our movements to meet socially acceptable standards. The next time you walk down the street, make mental contact with your pelvic region. Note whether or not you allow your hips to sway naturally with each stride; don't be surprised to find you are part of the stiff-hipped majority of Western society.

To counteract pelvic rigidity, do more aerobic activities and incorporate what I call the "pelvic swing" into your genital gymnastic routine. Like the PC muscle flex, the following exercise serves to increase genital awareness and tonicity, encourage energy to flow more freely into the pelvic region, and enhance the impact of the orgasm reflex. It will also have you moving through the world with a sexier, more liberated gait in no time!

Choose some music that will make you want to "move to the groove," then stand—ideally naked—in front of a full-length mirror. Spread your legs shoulders' width apart and flex your knees slightly, your feet pointing forward. Then find your center by granting yourself a moment of quiet introspection. Become aware of your breath. Note how it moves in, through, and out of your body. You are likely to discover that you are holding tension in your neck and shoulders. Take your time, be present, breathe deeply and with intent, and let the tension go.

When you feel mentally centered and physically ready, inhale deeply and thrust your hips with an exaggerated movement to the front; upon exhalation thrust them to the back. Repeat until you feel the muscles in your pelvic region start to relax, then change directions: with the same movements and breathing pattern, rock your hips from side to side.

Establish a rhythm by alternating between front and back and side to side until you feel ready to let loose; then make smooth, wide, circular patterns with your hips, first clockwise, then counterclockwise. Be aware of your breathing, and allow your entire body to ease into and flow with your movements. Don't be surprised if you find yourself having a good laugh. Smile back at yourself in the mirror, and have fun loosening up! If you have a Hula-Hoop, feel free to use that. Continue to gyrate, and it won't be long before you are working up a sweat. A minimum of ten minutes is sufficient, but the longer and the more often you do the pelvic swing, the more likely you are to reap the benefits that it provides both in and beyond the boudoir.

At the end of the pelvic swing, take a moment to become aware of the effects of the exercise. Lie down on your back, bend your knees, and plant your feet solidly on the floor, shoulders' width apart. Then, placing your hands on your lower abdomen, just above your pubic bone (fingers pointing toward your genitals), press your spinal column firmly against the floor. Make mental contact with your whole pelvic region before focusing on your genitals, where you are likely to notice a pleasant tingling sensation caused by the increased circulation.

Take advantage of this position to try the "sacral thump," another exercise that enhances circulation and reduces rigidity in the pelvic region—anorgasmic women find it especially helpful. On an exercise mat or similar surface, assume the same position as above—on your back with your knees bent and your feet on the floor. Then, pressing your spinal column firmly against the floor, lift your pelvis and let it fall, thumping your sacrum gently. Repeat until you are rewarded with a tingling sensation in the pelvic region.

When practiced regularly, the PC muscle flex, pelvic swing, and the sacral thump will keep the genitals toned and ready for action. Beyond facilitating ejaculation control in women and men (which the next chapters explore in detail), PC muscle tone and pelvic flexibility positively influence the orgasmic impact. The genital gym is an excellent way to warm up as you prepare to transcend.

CHAPTER 4

———o———

RIDING THE ORGASMIC WAVE:
MALE EJACULATION CONTROL

Is that a pistol in your pocket, or are you just happy to see me?

— Mae West

THE EMISSION OF SPERM into the outside world is still considered by many as the ultimate symbol of sexual superiority, prowess, and strength—in spite of the fact that it usually marks the abrupt end of any sexual encounter in which males are involved!

Deep pleasure is the raison d'être of the Paradise Found Sexual Ceremony, so in discussing male ejaculation control, my use of the terms "control" or "delay" in relation to male emission should not be confused with "denial." Today, as in historical times, men are often considered to be natural-born lovers, with innate sexual knowledge and skillfulness, and so there is little attention accorded to the subject of heightened male pleasures. But these pleasures, which stem from the techniques of ejaculation delay, are central to the elaboration of the Sexual Ceremony. While the techniques described within this chapter are male oriented, female partners are equally responsible for the positive evolution of the Sexual Ceremony and can learn how to help to execute some of them with their male partners—a shared act that can be as much an aphrodisiac as a bonding experience!

Controlling ejaculation, or riding the crest of the orgasmic wave until the conclusive orgasm, permits men to mount sexual tension to higher, more ecstatic degrees over long periods of ever-more-pleasurable stimulation and results in the enhancement of all sensory pleasures, including orgasms. Its related counterpart, the internal orgasm, is hailed not only for instilling heightened degrees of sexual satisfaction and avoiding the "little death" but also for the fact that it permits men to obtain multiorgasmic equality with their female counterparts. This would seem to be reason enough for every Western male to embark upon an alternative-orgasm mission, but most men continue to believe that their relatively fast ejaculation is the pinnacle of the sexual experience and that multi-orgasmic pleasures are the sole domain of the uninhibited, sexually experienced woman.

As described in the chapter "The Genital Gym: Strengthening the Pubococcygeal Muscle," learning to control and strengthen the pubococcygeal (PC) muscle is indispensable to the ability to delay the ejaculation reflex. Along with a skilled administration of full-body sensations, PC muscle control also enhances excitement throughout the pleasurably long period of arousal that constitutes the Paradise Found Sexual Ceremony.

THE END?: EJACULATION CONTROL RECONSIDERED

Practitioners of the Tao of Loving consider a man's capacity to control the ejaculation reflex as crucial to the mutual attainment of sexual satisfaction. Devotees of Tantric ritual sex, which is called Yoni Puja, or "the Cult of the Vagina," also place an emphasis on the importance of ejaculation delay for enhanced pleasure—of benefit to the physical as well as spiritual well-being of both partners.

After the art of meditation, both Tantrists and Taoists hail ejaculation control as the most immediate path to transcendental pleasures and spiritual illumination. This is in striking contrast to the Judeo-Christian patriarchs, who, in order to come closer to God, propagated the idea that abstinence is the only way to avoid wasteful, unholy ejaculations.

Judeo-Christian superiors-cum-saints understood only part of the issue. It is a fact that in avoiding ejaculation, men can avoid its exhausting side effects. Even though a single emission may seem insignificant, the average amount being only one or two teaspoons of fluid, it contains anywhere from 50 to 250 million sperm, all leaving the body at an average speed of 28 miles per hour (45 kilometers per hour)! This represents an astronomical dispersion of creative energy potential and helps to explain why men often demand immediate rest following ejaculation. This aftereffect of sex, sometimes called "the little death," is no doubt the reason why sperm is considered a precious force not to be wasted by virtually every culture—pornography notwithstanding.

The ultimate goal of the techniques of ejaculation control developed by both the Tantrists in India and the Taoists in China was the internal orgasm, or the disassociation of the orgasm and ejaculation reflexes (not to be confused with internal ejaculation). Usually, the ejaculation reflex occurs when semen, containing sperm and male hormones such as testosterone, exits the prostate gland and fills the urethral canal. During an internal orgasm, the man restrains this reflex, augmenting the ecstatic sensations of orgasm that are generated in part by the vibration, or fluttering, of the prostate gland. These sensations can be experienced over and over again during prolonged periods of arousal, as long as the ejaculation reflex is kept under control and seminal fluid is not allowed to exit the prostate gland and move toward the urethral opening. To ride the crest of the orgasmic wave, rather than succumb to the ejaculation reflex, is the essence of the internal orgasm. It is also the foundation of the multiple orgasm, or the "valley orgasm," as the Taoists poetically describe it. Men who learn to experience multiple internal orgasms describe the satiating pleasures they provide in terms similar to those used by multiorgasmic women.

Being that the topic of internal orgasm merits more attention than space here allows, this chapter concentrates on the techniques that allow men to control the ejaculation reflex, which is essential to the elaboration of the Paradise Found Sexual Ceremony (except for female-to-female encounters). Most of these techniques are directly related to the Taoist and Tantric disciplines of internal emission, so with diligent practice, it is not unlikely that men will eventually experience the ecstatic effects of the internal orgasm. Those who wish to master the techniques of internal orgasm to perfection should consider seeking guidance from a skilled master in the Tantric or Taoist arts of loving.

THE POINT OF NO RETURN

To practice the methods of male ejaculation control, men must learn to recognize and respond to the sensations that lead up to what is known as "the point of no return," as Dr. William Masters and Virginia Johnson named it in the 1970s. The first phase of the orgasm reflex is signaled when the sperm exit the testicles and begin their outward journey. The second phase is signaled when the seminal fluid enters the prostate gland. Its exit from the prostate gland, filling the urethral canal, puts the prostate gland under pressure and prompts the ejaculation reflex.

Learning to recognize the signs and sensations that lead up to the point of no return is crucial to the evolution of the Sexual Ceremony. Before ejaculation, a muscle known as the cremaster, located within the scrotum, contracts involuntarily, causing the interior walls of the scrotum to retract into the inner walls of the pelvic area. This pulls the testicles upward toward the body—one visible sign of imminent ejaculation. If lovers do not heed this warning sign, the sperm will continue their outward journey. Once they exit the prostate gland, it is next to impossible to prevent the emission of seminal fluid into the outside world.

The clear, slippery fluid colloquially known as pre-cum is another sign of imminent ejaculation. Some men emit this fluid long before they actually ejaculate, but either way its manifestation is a clear indication of a heightened degree of arousal. Lovers must gauge the administration of sensations in such a way as to avoid taking an aroused partner over the edge before the Sexual Ceremony is due to end.

Excitement is also indicated by changes in breathing patterns. Some men begin to breathe more rapidly, taking shallow breaths. Some men become more vocal as their pleasure deepens. This being said, other men silently hold their breath! The outward signs of imminent ejaculation vary from man to man, so the better lovers get to know each other, the more adept they will be at reading each other's body language. Verbal communication is one of the most effective ways for a highly aroused man to avoid having his partner involuntarily push him over the edge of ecstasy, bringing the ceremony to a premature end.

Partake in solo masturbation rituals, men, to learn to avoid the point of no return. No matter the method you use, always remember to stay in the moment and focus your thoughts on the exhilarating sensations that the flux of the sexual energy in the genitals incites. (In other words, don't follow the common practice of distracting yourself with non-erotic thoughts!) Be aware of your breathing: breathe with deep, steady inhalations and exhalations. This encourages the flow of fresh, oxygenated blood throughout the entire body, enhancing your pleasure as well as your sense of mental presence and clarity, which is essential to the techniques of ejaculation control. And remember not to judge or put yourself under pressure to "perform." With ecstatic practice, you are guaranteed to become a master of the delights of delay. During the solo masturbation ritual make a point to "peak," that is, to repeatedly push your orgasmic limit but without going over the edge. Peaking allows you to mount sexual tension gradually and to great heights.

Once you have learned to recognize and respond effectively to your body's built-in ejaculation messenger, you will be able to share the delights of delay in the Paradise Found Sexual Ceremony. When the orgasmic wave is finally permitted to flow and ebb, the radical benefits of delay, in comparison to the fleeting gratification of fast PGO sex, will be evident.

INTERNAL EMISSION

As men begin to master the following techniques, emission may occur not only externally but also internally; that is, semen will not exit the body through the urethral opening. Men may experience sensations that are similar to those they feel when they orgasm in association with the emission of semen, but instead of the fluid exiting the body, it is diverted from the prostate and goes directly into the bladder. The erection will subside, and before the Sexual Ceremony can resume, the man will be obliged to submit to a refractory (or rest) period, exactly as if he had ejaculated externally.

The results of internal emission can be observed: urinate directly afterward into a transparent container, and you will immediately note the cloudiness of your urine, caused by the presence of semen. Internal emission does not present any health risks or other side effects, but it is not the goal of ejaculation control.

AN INVITATION INTO POTENT PLEASURE SECRETS

Mastering the Pelvic Lock
The techniques of ejaculation control demand a toned PC muscle.

All of the techniques of ejaculation control are to be practiced in coordination with the pelvic lock—the conscious contraction of the PC and the sphincter muscles described as the "PC muscle flex" in the chapter "The Genital Gym: Strengthening the Pubococcygeal Muscle." Men who master the manual techniques in coordination with the pelvic lock may eventually find that executing only the pelvic lock (albeit with acute mental awareness and controlled breathing patterns) will often suffice to inhibit the ejaculation reflex. Refining your skills to this degree has a great advantage—that of leaving your hands free to perform other tantalizing tasks!

Practice the PC muscle flex regularly, and, over time and with practice, avoiding the point of no return will become as simple as refocusing one's thoughts. Men, to magnify the effects of the pelvic lock, spread your legs wide apart when you tighten the PC and sphincter; this will serve to minimize the pressure that the PC and sphincter muscles usually apply to the prostate and to the vas deferens, the duct that propels semen from the testicles through the male genital organ system, just before ejaculation.

Vibrating with the Finger Lock
Like the pelvic lock, the finger lock manipulates the vas deferens, but it does so through direct pressure. The ancient Taoist master Lu the Immortal ordered his disciples to swear an oath that they would not divulge the potent secret of this technique to the uninitiated. In accordance with the mission of this book, please consider this an initiation, and feel free to divulge!

When executed skillfully, the finger lock inhibits the reflexive contractions of the vas deferens, preventing the outward journey of seminal fluid during both the first and second phases of the orgasm. The portion of the vas deferens that we are concerned with corresponds to an acupuncture point, which is located in the perineal wall, just in front of the anus. Composed of strong, smooth muscles,

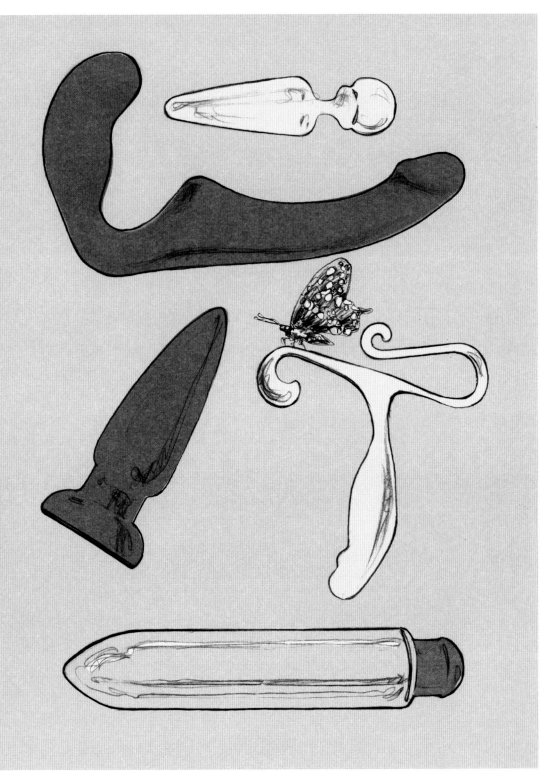

PLATE V IMPLEMENTS FOR PENETRATION

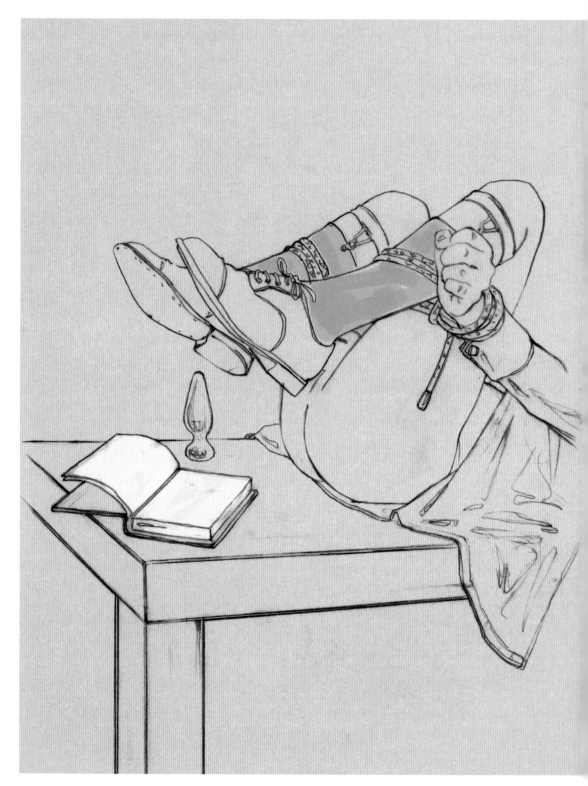

PLATE VI BONDAGE SESSION WITH ANAL PLEASURE

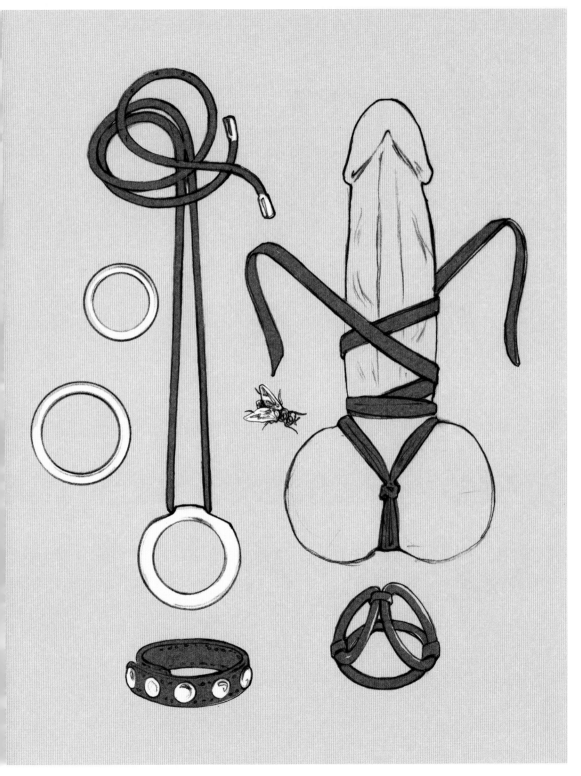

PLATE VII INSTRUMENTS FOR MALE EJACULATION CONTROL

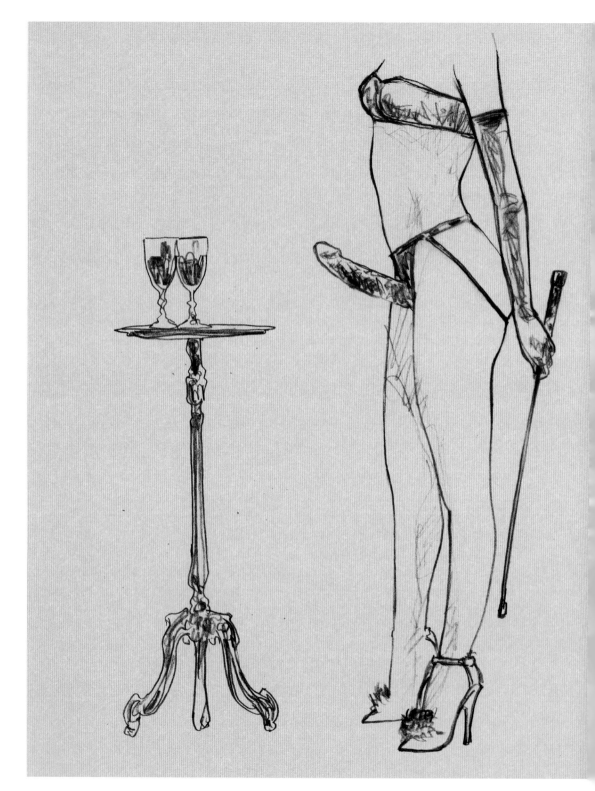

PLATE VIII ROLE-REVERSAL SESSION WITH STRAP-ON DILETTO

the vas deferens's ridged, tubular shape is approximately ⅛ of an inch (3 millimeters) in diameter.

Men, as soon as you (or your partner) perceive a sign of imminent ejaculation, press the area in front of the anus firmly with the fingers until the fingertips sink approximately one knuckle deep into the engorged tissues. This procedure, which inhibits emission, can also be used to divert the ejaculate fluid back into the prostatic region (just in the nick of time!). Some men find that using the knuckles rather than the fingertips provides a deeper degree of pressure. Folding the knees up to the chest may also facilitate your reaching this portion of the perineum. With practice, the position and the means that work best for each individual will be revealed.

To ride the crest of the orgasmic wave for as long as you possibly can, keep from ejaculating by concentrating on the sensations evoked by applying pressure to the vas deferens through the perineal wall. Don't be surprised if you find yourself vibrating to the vigorous pulsations and ecstatic sensations that are produced by the prostate gland during orgasm, but without actually emitting fluid. This is the essence of internal and multiple male orgasms! Breathe deeply, continue to execute the pelvic lock in coordination with the finger lock, and enjoy the ecstatic sensations.

To ensure even more control over the ejaculation reflex, many ancient Taoist texts encourage assuming the hysterical arch, which I call the "control arch" in reference to male lovers: arch your back like a female porn star, clench your teeth, and close your eyes, elongating your neck and pressing your tongue hard against your upper palate. The control arch short-circuits blood flow to the genitals and inhibits orgasm; while it works to the disadvantage of women, in the context of male ejaculation control, this position greatly benefits both ceremonial partners.

The Taoist master Tung recommended another control technique: The man should close his eyes and focus on the sensations. Pressing his tongue against the roof of his mouth, he should bend his back and stretch his neck. Opening his nostrils wide and drawing back his shoulders, he should then close his mouth and draw in his breath through his nostrils. This will stop him from ejaculating and cause his semen to ascend upward.

One of my favorite Taoist lessons involves another acupuncture point: the *pin yi*, which is located in the middle of the right breast, approximately 2 to 3 inches (5 to 7 centimeters) above the nipple. Pinpoint the location of this sensitive zone within a solo masturbation ritual by applying firm, direct pressure to the area with one or two fingertips. Once you find your pin yi and are illuminated by its power to help you "short-circuit" your emission, enlighten your partner!

Incorporate into your own style any of the gestures that have been explored thus far. By facilitating your ability to delay ejaculation, they will help to make the shared pleasures of your journey into the heights of the now potentially transcendent sexual dimension all the more exciting and fulfilling!

Sharing the Ball Lock

Another manual technique is called the ball lock, which can be employed by the man in question or his partner. As soon as the scrotum begins to draw up close to the body, encircle the entire portion of the scrotum that lies closest to the base of the penis and the perineum with the thumb and forefinger. Carefully trapped in this ringlike grip, the scrotum can be drawn downward and away from the body, inhibiting the sperm from exiting the testicles. Depending on the size of your scrotal sack, you may need to draw the testicles down one at a time. Once the risk of ejaculation has passed, the sensitive skin of the scrotum, now stretched tightly around the testicles, can be licked, sucked, scratched, tickled, and caressed to your delight. Your partner must just be careful of the delicate skin of the scrotum and take great care to avoid pushing the testicles upward toward the body; as any man can tell, it will inflict excruciating pain!

Perfecting the Squeeze Method
The squeeze method is a Taoist and Tantric technique that is commonly prescribed by sex therapists to retrain patients who suffer from premature ejaculation. The technique is performed on the head of the penis as soon as the first sign of the point of no return is signaled. Apply decisive, direct pressure with the thumb and forefinger just below the ridge of the glans. The technique is more effective if pressure is applied only at the front and back of the penis, not at the sides. Once you have perfected the gesture, the same degree of pressure may be applied at the very base of the shaft, again at the front and back, not at the sides. By redirecting the point of pressure from the base of the gland to the base of the shaft, the squeeze method can also be practiced during penetration.

TO EJACULATE OR NOT TO EJACULATE?

At this point, most of you are probably wondering if the Paradise Found Sexual Ceremony is anti-male ejaculation, and the answer is no, of course not! Male partners who learn to control their ejaculation reflex and peak skillfully can ride the crest of the orgasmic wave over and over again throughout the ceremony. When they finally do allow themselves to surpass the point of no return, whether they actually ejaculate or not, earth-shattering effects are guaranteed.

Regulating ejaculation is crucial for shaping the phases of the Sexual Ceremony. For example, if partners intend to play for three hours, which is the ideal minimum, men should try to refrain from ejaculating until the very end. If the ceremony is organized to last more than three hours, men need to regulate emission in such a way as to permit the ceremony's harmonious evolution. But while it is ideal that emission occur at the end of the ritual, any time over-arousal results in emission, consider it an intermission in the Sexual Ceremony—enjoy taking care of each other in different ways. Once the refractory period has passed and the male partner becomes receptive to genital or full-body stimulation again, the ceremony can be resumed.

Men, if at any time you feel the point of no return approaching, feel free to perform the techniques of ejaculation control that you have found most effective, or ask your partner to do so. Your partner's attention should also shift from your genitals to a less-sensitive erogenous zone of your body until direct genital contact can be resumed without compromising the ceremony's evolution. When peaking in tandem, lovers should guide each other both verbally and physically, without shame or inhibition, while remaining aware of each other's levels of arousal. Backing off may be as simple as slowing down or changing the rhythm of stimulation and the tools or techniques used to provide sensations.

This is also an excellent time for partners to alternate between the roles of provider and receiver of sensations. Remember that overemphasis upon the male genitals is likely to make for a fleeting sexual exchange, while sharing pleasures that alternate between genital and extra-genital stimulation generates the ecstatic essence of the ceremony.

DO NOT LET YOUR SPIRIT SUFFER!

The masters of the ancient arts of loving learned to enjoy the benefits of orgasm without necessarily ejaculating and recommended refraining from too-frequent emission as a way to greater health as well as pleasure. Ejaculating more than once per day has a draining effect on a man's energy and also decreases the impact of the pleasures that each consecutive orgasm will provide over the course of the same day.

The Taoists maintain that frequent male emission causes the libido to dwindle, and it is one of the reasons that they associated ejaculation control with increased desire as well as enhanced pleasure. The Tao of Loving proposes ejaculating only two or three times out of ten encounters—a challenge for most unless one is skilled in the technique of internal orgasm. Taoist master of the Han dynasty Wu Hsien suggested that man should practice "retention for at least five-thousand love strokes before ejaculating, as then his whole being will become potentized." According to Master Wu Hsien, the principal concern of a male practitioner of the Tao of Loving should be to bring his female partner to orgasm as frequently as possible, taking advantage of the sexual vibration generated by his female partner's pleasure by absorbing yin, or female energy, from her genitals with his "jade stalk."

Taoist masters encourage men to externalize emission from time to time in order to avoid "overheating" the organism and compromising the overall health benefits that the sexual union provides and the fortitude of the sperm. Yet when Taoist males are deprived of the company of partners, they are encouraged to masturbate to the point of ejaculation more frequently, in order to avoid the prolonged retention of ejaculate fluid blocking the flow of energy, or chi, that flows more readily during partner sex.

An ancient Chinese medical manual declares that "man cannot do without woman, and woman cannot do without man. If a man does not make love with a woman for a long period of time, his mind will grow very unmanageable. If this happens, his spirit will suffer, and if the spirit suffers, then his span of life will be shortened."

Men, whether you prefer men, women, or both—do not let your spirit suffer! There are many tools and techniques to enhance your skills and pleasures. Dildos and vibrators, essentially prosthetic penises, bestow delights that serve to prolong the Sexual Ceremony, building sexual tension and pleasure; tools such as cock rings can be used to facilitate the joys of peaking and augment the mutual benefits of ejaculation delay.

COCK RINGS: FOR EXTRA-PLEASURABLE PLAYTIME

Cock rings and cock-and-ball rings serve to delay ejaculation and have the added benefit of leaving the man's hands free to provide other pleasures (see plate VII, page 119). Some men find it impossible to ejaculate while cock rings are in place, and this is the principal reason why I mention these tools in the context of ejaculation control. When using a cock ring, men are likely to experience the pleasurable fluttering of the prostate gland that is inherent to the internal orgasm. The related topic of tying the male genitals is explored in the chapter "Abandon Yourself: Erotic Restraints."

Made from a myriad of materials, from metal to leather, wood, carved stone, glass, rubber, plastic, and just about anything else that can take the shape of a ring, cock rings add an aesthetically pleasing touch to playtime. Some men prefer leather and rubber cock rings that have snaps to allow for easy removal, but cock rings made in rigid materials are equally effective and can be worn without creating any degree of discomfort, as long as they fit properly.

Smaller-diameter cock rings can be worn anywhere along the shaft of the penis. Those that fit snugly on the upper and lower areas of the shaft can be used to execute variations on the squeeze method. Rings in larger diameters are designed to constrict both the base of the penis and the entirety of the scrotal sack, essentially executing a combination of the squeeze method at the base of the penis and the ball lock. More commonly known as cock-and-ball rings, these are more effective in delaying ejaculation than rings that fit along the shaft. Size is important in cock rings: a ring that is too big will do very little to enhance a man's pleasure or ability to control ejaculation, and a ring that is too small risks compromising the flow of blood into the penis.

Being that cock rings are rarely sold with instructions for their correct use, many men are nervous about the possibility of damaging their "family jewels" and refrain from exploring their potential. The basic rule of thumb is as follows: smaller-diameter cock rings can be put in place *after* a full erection is attained, but cock-and-ball rings should be put in place *before* the penis is fully erect. It will otherwise be next to impossible to accomplish the task.

Employing a rigid cock-and-ball ring can be awkward, if not impossible, unless you know the following tips: Remember that the penis must not be fully erect. Hold the ring in one hand and pull the testicles through its center one by one with the other hand. Once the scrotal sac is within its grip, the head and then the entire shaft of the penis can be pulled through the ring. Once the ring is in place, it should fit snugly around the scrotum and the base of the shaft of the penis. The size of the ring should be more or less right if there is space enough to slide the index and middle fingers between the ring and the penis before complete erection is obtained. Once the penis is fully erect, this will no longer be possible.

The ring should create a pleasant sense of constriction but no feeling of discomfort. When the scrotum and base of the shaft are enclosed in the grip of a cock-and-ball ring, once the penis reaches full erection, it is obliged to remain erect for as long as stimulation continues. The vas deferens is put under pressure while the blood that races into the genitals during arousal is inhibited from flowing back out again, resulting in harder, more enduring erections.

Men, once your penis and/or scrotum is in the grip of a cock ring, it is essential to pay close attention to the sensations caused by constriction, especially if it is the first time that you have used a ring. If you prefer a tighter fit, it is important to ensure that the blood flow to the area is not entirely constrained, especially over extended periods of play. Neither your penis nor the scrotum should go cold, numb, or turn worrisome shades of blue! If they do, the ring is too tight and it has been in place for too long.

You may be anxious about getting "trapped" in a cock ring. Worry not: once your erection subsides, or you or your partner make it subside by refraining from direct stimulation, the ring will slide off easily. If you wish to speed up the process, rinse your genitals with cold water.

The recommended time limit for wearing a cock ring is about twenty minutes, but it actually depends on the degree to which the genitals are constricted. Listen to your body and learn your own limits by starting out slowly and trying different kinds and sizes of rings. Some men like to wear cock rings for much longer periods, even for an entire evening out on the town. As long the rings are not too tight, this is safe, but long-term wear should be left to experienced cock-ring aficionados. But do keep in mind that if you decide to wear your cock ring beyond the boudoir, the device is likely to keep the penis in slight erection, even for an entire evening, and the effects are likely to be noticed if you are wearing close-fitting clothing or trousers made in fine fabrics.

DELIGHTS OF THE PROSTHETIC PENIS

In the Paradise Found Sexual Ceremony, a dildo, or the term that I prefer, a diletto, can stand in for the actual penis whenever over-arousal risks triggering the ejaculation reflex and therefore potentially halting the progression of the ritual. I like the word "diletto," derived from the Italian verb *dilettare*, because of its meaning: to delight, amuse, and give pleasure. I use "diletto" to describe any object used as a substitute for the penis, including vibrators. By permitting lovers to engage in longer intervals of penetration, dilettos further enhance the delights of delay. They allow over-aroused men to back off while continuing to provide their partners with the delights of penetration. Dilettos not only ease the demands placed upon the male member over lengthy rituals but provide both vaginal and anal stimulation. And the fact that dilettos endow women with the power to penetrate, and even be penetrated in the absence of a male partner, is obviously not something to undervalue!

In Tantric and Taoist practices, dilettos were used to help prolong sexual rituals. Ancient Eastern art and literature commonly portray their ecstatically profane and highly sacred purpose in detail. The predecessors of the modern-day diletto were first made in stone and iron, and a few have been found to date as far back as 28,000 years before the birth of Christ. In Africa, the finest dilettos were made of ivory. In ancient Greece and Rome, they were made of a variety of materials, from wood and ceramic to blown glass, silver, and even gold. In Arabian and Polynesian cultures, dilettos literally grew on trees. In *The Arabian Nights*, a passage is dedicated to the wonders of the banana:

"O bananas, of soft and smooth skins which dilate the eyes of young girls . . . you alone among fruits are endowed with a pitying heart, O consolers of widows and divorced women."

The *Kama Sutra* also suggests the use of "natural" dildos. Bananas are mentioned, as well as carrots, cucumbers, and gourds. If you are feeling gourmand and decide to use produce that resembles the erect lingam as part of your play, protect yourself from exposure to toxins by dressing it with a condom. Unless the fruits and vegetables were organically grown, you can be certain that their surfaces contain traces of toxic pesticides.

But remember: no matter what they are made of, dilettos used for anal stimulation should *never* be then used for vaginal pleasures unless they are dressed with a fresh condom after each phase of penetration. It is highly recommended that lovers designate one diletto for vaginal pleasuring and another one specifically to anal stimulation.

The condom rule also applies to any modern-day diletto that is made of rubber, latex, silicone, or other flexible plastics. Even though these materials emulate the penis better than harder materials, they are porous and extremely difficult to sanitize. They also have a tendency to degrade over time. The best way to prolong their durability and ensure that they do not provoke irritations and infections is to dress them with condoms. Note that silicone-based lubricants deteriorate silicone sex tools over time, so the use of water- or glycerine-based lubricants is highly advised.

Flexible plastic dilettos should never be used without a condom unless they are explicitly declared body safe, as they are otherwise more than likely to contain phthalates, a chemical compound that is added to plastic to render it flexible. Also found in soft plastic toys for children, phthalates have been linked to birth defects, dangerous alterations in hormone levels, and damage to the liver, testicles, and other organs.

A Sexual Ally
Some men may consider dilettos or vibrators to be a threat to their own sexuality. More often than not this is due to the implements' typically over-endowed dimensions as well as their infinite power to please. Most male-oriented sex suppliers carry a range of extra-large dilettos that would effectively make 99.9 percent of the male population feel inadequate! But these huge prosthetics are rarely modeled after real penises (nor are they the best sellers). But can a tool really be considered a threat to a relationship? After all, nothing can replace the energy exchange that is generated between two living, loving, physical entities, and men may certainly choose a diletto whose dimensions enable it to be more an ally than an enemy.

Models that are designed to wear with harnesses are known as strap-ons (see plate VIII, page 120), and they endow women with the power to penetrate. Double dilettos, on the other hand, can be used by either gender, and they have the advantage of allowing lovers to penetrate while they are simultaneously being penetrated. Some double dilettos are designed specifically for women, with one end that fits into the vagina. Whenever possible, women should wear these in combination with a harness to allow for a greater degree of comfort and control, and which also frees hands to roam. "Strapping-on" creates a reversal in roles—the woman becomes the penetrator and the male becomes the "penetratee"—which is likely to intimidate men who have not been initiated into the pleasures of anal sex; my advice to partners is to discuss the use of strap-on dilettos before making use of them.

The Vibrating Cousin
Vibrators, the vibrating cousin of the diletto, tend to be marketed with solitary women in mind, but their power to intensify the impact of shared sexual pleasures should not be underestimated. Some vibrators, however, are designed for clitoral stimulation and as such are not meant to be inserted into the body. I personally prefer and will here refer to those that can be used exactly like dilettos, to provide both vaginal and anal pleasures as well as clitoral delights. Taking an erotic intermission in the sexual ceremony and watching a lover writhe to the pulse of a vibrating lingam is indisputably arousing. Hand-held mirrors can be used to permit partners to share the vision.

No matter the tools or the techniques employed to facilitate ejaculation control, once men have learned to recognize and respond effectively to their point of no return, they can engage in extensive periods of stimulation and heighten their satisfaction!

CHAPTER 5

───── o ─────

NAVIGATING THE SACRED RIVER:
FEMALE EMISSIONS

Sex is a natural function. You can't make it happen,
but you can teach people to let it happen.

— Dr. William H. Masters

THE PHENOMENON OF ejaculation was considered to be the greatest difference between male and female sexual functions until the beginning of the 1980s, when the female prostate and its palpable manifestation, the G-spot, were rediscovered and their connection to female emission scientifically proven.

Yet in spite of the clinical research, laboratory testing, and case studies from the past thirty years, female ejaculation and the related but very different jets or streams of "squirting" continue to be a topic of controversy. The facts, however, are that fluid produced in the female prostate during heightened states of arousal contains biochemical components comparable to those in semen, including prostate-specific antigen (PSA) which happens to be produced in only one other gland in the human body: the male prostate! The fluids from ejaculation and squirting exit the body, just as male ejaculate does, via the urethral canal. Misinformed lovers commonly mistake female squirting for urine; this misperception can lead to debilitating feelings of shame in women and confusion in men.

Some researchers and doctors tiptoe around the topic by maintaining that women once had the ability to ejaculate, but as it merely served an antibacterial function in reproduction, the organ responsible for ejaculation atrophied with the advent of modern hygiene. Many medical professionals continue to deny scientific evidence altogether. This has led to the acute lack of accurate public information about female emissions, which in turn not only propagates the female ejaculation taboo but also leads perfectly healthy women to seek surgical "cures" for squirting, which was diagnosed as coital incontinence in the 1950s.

The Paradise Found Sexual Ceremony brings lovers into contact with the whole of their sexual beings—as men explore heightened pleasure through prostate stimulation and the delights of delay, women discover entirely new horizons of pleasure when their G-spot awakens. But it is important to keep in mind that, like any journey in life, the sexual path is the destination: women, seek G-spot orgasms and create the conditions to prompt emissions, but don't let that goal keep you from enjoying every other source of pleasure that you will experience along the way.

THE FLOOD OF VENUS

Female emissions, represented in ancient art, artifacts, architecture, and literature throughout all cultures, is often depicted or described as a river or stream flowing from the female genitals. Poetic names from ancient literature reflect the positive manner in which the phenomenon was viewed: the flood of Venus, the elixir of life, the sacred river, the nectar of the gods, and the lotus nectar. The *Kama Sutra* speaks of female emissions in terms of "seed that . . . continues to fall from the beginning of the sexual union to its end." The elixir was renowned by the Taoists for its legendary ability to reverse the aging process. Skilled lovers in sixteenth-century Japan collected the aphrodisiacal cocktail in bowls designed specifically to capture its flux. Those who consumed the fluid felt all the happier and more rejuvenated. This may in part be explained by the traces of the neurotransmitter serotonin that female emission contains.

Other cultures known to have considered female emission as an essential aspect of female pleasure were the Tantrists, the ancient Greeks and Romans, the Celts, the Cherokee Indians in North America, and the Trukese of the Coral Islands in the South Pacific; in all of these societies, female emissions were viewed as symbols of woman's "masculine" side, a perspective that rendered women sexually equal to men.

A SOURCE OF UNEQUALED PLEASURE

The generation of prostate fluid is the body's involuntary physiological response to arousal, and nothing can prevent the intricate network of ducts and glands that compose the female prostate, the largest of which is known as the Skene's glands, from producing this fluid. But over the centuries, like the female orgasm itself, this biological response was repressed to the point that the majority of women essentially have "forgotten" how to ejaculate! However, most highly aroused women emit imperceptible quantities of prostate fluid through the urethral opening before, during, and after orgasm. Those who "remember" how to ejaculate and abandon themselves to the sensations that lead up to ejaculation may also "squirt"—clinical reports giving the amount of fluid as between 1 and 3 ounces (25 and 100 milliliters)! Labeled *femmes fontaines*, literally "fountain ladies," by the French psychologist Frédérique Gruyer in 1984, these women are proof that the female prostate has not atrophied; they constitute, however, a mere 6 to 8 percent of the female population today.

Every sexually mature woman has a prostate and paraurethral glands that produce and store prostate fluid (even if most anatomical charts for the female genital system still fail to represent these). Theoretically, any woman can learn to create the conditions for ejaculation and squirting and revel in the heightened degrees of sexual satisfaction that they excite—and the empowering sense of equality that accompanies emission. We may therefore conclude that what women seem to be missing, more than anything else, are equally informed, sufficiently liberated, and well-skilled partners!

Fast PGO sex does not promote female emissions, while the Paradise Found Sexual Ceremony, with its slow building of sexual tension, provides lovers with the perfect opportunity to explore the ecstatic powers of the G-spot and encourage the flow of female fluids. The prime conditions are extensive periods of stimulation, heightened degrees of arousal, direct G-spot stimulation, multiple orgasms, lack of inhibition, and being truly attracted to and confident with one's partner, which instills a sense of ease and openness to what may come. Lovers who revel in the pleasures that lead to female emissions consider the G-spot to be the source of unequaled delight and emission to be a highlight of their sexual endeavors, as well as the most generously ecstatic way for a woman to thank her partner for worshipping her to such an extent.

Female ejaculate fluid has the look and consistency of semen, while squirt is noted for its clarity and has the consistency of water. Its distinct perfume is most commonly described as the refreshing smell of spring rain, but some women also report their emissions as having salty sea tones, floral scents, or earthy undertones of amber, musk, or moss. These variations are determined in part by variations in diet. The transparency of squirt may vary and even become slightly cloudy with approaching menstruation. Women, if you eventually revitalize your capacity to squirt, ask your lover to collect some of the liquid that you emit in a glass or bowl as it leaves your body. Smell and even taste it just as our ancient ancestors did, and invite your partner to do the same. This can be an extremely exciting aspect of the Sexual Ceremony (but obviously one that should only be shared by lovers who have a safe fluid-exchange agreement).

Facilitate your heavenly delight by playing on surfaces that will not be damaged by liquids and protecting those that could be damaged with towels. Consider investing in a latex sheet. Designed to fit various sizes of mattresses, it can be purchased online and in most sex shops. Whether you are a novice to G-spot stimulation or an experienced femme fontaine, being worried about making a mess will hold you back from abandoning yourself to the pleasures of G-spot stimulation.

AWAKENING THE G-SPOT

Awakening the G-spot takes blissful time and a relaxed state of mind and body, so it's best to initiate this kind of exploration when you have the time and energy to build sexual tension to the heights. And, of course, leave expectations that lead to performance-pressure out of the boudoir. Even the most insensitive, sleepy, or oversensitized G-spot can be coaxed to sweet reception, if sufficient care and attention are dedicated to "retraining" it to respond positively to direct contact.

Note that the G-spot is connected to the powerful pelvic splanchnic nerve, and so stimulating the area may evoke more emotional responses than those derived through clitoral stimulation. It is for this reason that Tantric lovers associate G-spot stimulation with the opening of the heart chakra, and the foundation of intimate bonds between partners.

Women, that means that if you are a novice to the effects of G-spot stimulation, you may wish to explore the zone on your own first. A solo masturbation ritual will help you get to know your G-spot and permit those who suffer from G-spot numbness, oversensitivity, or related anxiety to awaken the sensitive area gradually and experience the deep degrees of satisfaction it can and should provide. Once you feel comfortable with G-spot stimulation on your own, invite your lover to help navigate your sacred river.

Most informed lovers are more than willing to share in the mutual delights of G-spot stimulation and female ejaculation, but some men may initially fear that their own pleasure will dissipate in the time that it takes to awaken the G-spot and provoke emission. Others may be intimidated by women's potential to ejaculate and squirt repeatedly without compromising their sexual fulfillment or their desire. But G-spot stimulation can only augment the male partner's pleasure, as the Paradise Found Sexual Ceremony transpires over extended periods of arousal in which both partners alternately provide and receive sensations, both genitally and extra-genitally oriented. In addition, if the male partner is skilled in the techniques of ejaculation control, he will have plenty of occasions to reach the pinnacles of his own pleasure—keep in mind that the most effective aphrodisiac is the pleasure that we provide.

If you are an experienced femme fontaine, never take an unknowing lover by surprise, but rather participate directly in the dismantling of the female emission taboo by preparing him or her in advance. Guiding your partner lovingly, especially in a ritualized context that is conducive to mutual arousal, will reinforce your intimate bond while allowing your partner to develop the sexual skills that call the G-spot into action.

Stroking the G-spot before the physical signs of female arousal have fully manifested is likely to cause more discomfort than pleasure, while climaxing, either clitorally or via the A-spot (the zone that lies deep within the vaginal canal near the cervix) increases the G-spot's receptivity to touch, as the female prostate becomes engorged with ejaculate fluid. Envision the highly sensitive G-spot as the delta of the sacred river that originates in the prostate. You must awaken the receptivity of the G-spot in order to eventually encourage the emission of its sacred fluids.

EMBRACING THE SENSATIONS

A woman who is a novice to the G-spot's powers should orgasm, then "peak" (repeatedly push one's orgasmic limit without cumming) before making direct contact with the highly sensitive area. The more charged with sexual vibration, the greater her receptivity to any form of stimulation. As soon as the warm, soft interiors of the vaginal canal are well lubricated and the female genitals begin to swell with pleasure, the G-spot will become more turgid and thus easier to locate. Some lovers confuse the wetness that high levels of sexual arousal generate in the vagina with female ejaculation, but remember that female emissions do not exit the body through the vaginal opening but directly through the urethral opening. However, just like the swelling of the G-spot, vaginal lubrication indicates that the G-spot is receptive to touch and signals that ejaculate fluid is beginning to build inside the female prostate.

Once arousal has deepened and the genitals have become engorged with excitement, great attention can be dedicated to the G-spot. For a novice, the fingers are the best method for understanding the zone, whether you are a woman exploring her own G-spot in a solo masturbation ritual or the partner of a woman.

Feel for a slightly raised mass of tissue approximately the size and shape of an almond on the anterior wall of the vagina, close to the vaginal opening. Explore its contours and then stroke it, gradually increasing the pressure. The pressure you apply should never generate discomfort. Meditate on the G-spot: Focus your full attention on the area and experiment with the range of sensations it provides.

Women, breathe deeply and with intention into these sensations as they gradually build, and the pleasure will be accompanied by an elevated state of relaxation and mental clarity. During this erotic meditation, your sensory awareness will become ever more acute—augmenting your perception of pleasure and allowing the sensations to radiate from the genitals to the extremities of the body. Body, mind, and spirit will benefit.

Note that simply sliding one or two fingers into the vagina will not call the G-spot into action; the area responds to direct and persistent contact. Once the G-spot's responses become familiar, try another object—a partner's penis or fingers, a diletto, or what is commonly known as a G-spotter.

Women, if your pleasure builds to the point of a G-spot orgasm, embrace its unequaled sensations. If, on the other hand, a clitoral orgasm rises on your sexually charged horizon, keep from succumbing to its pleasures—peak and surf its crest, but try to back off before the orgasmic wave actually breaks. This will prompt a surge of ejaculate fluid in the prostate while driving the sexual tension even higher. After all, patience is a virtue; peaking is not a denial of your pleasures but an enhancement in the context of extended playtime, and the results are likely to push you over the edge of ecstasy.

If your partner uses his penis or his or her fingers to penetrate you, he or she will perceive the various degrees of sensation that the vagina's tensing, gentle pushing, and relaxing will provide. This warm, wet genital embrace has the added advantage of enhancing your partner's levels of excitement as well as yours. But note that, given the length of time needed to generate the ecstatic conditions that build up ejaculate fluid within the female prostate and provoke its emission, a man must be careful to avoid passing "the point of no return." Consider that even an experienced femme fontaine may require anywhere from thirty to forty minutes to completely awaken the G-spot and attain the degrees of arousal that lead to emission.

This holds particularly true when she has not engaged in sexual contact for some time.

Deep thrusts provide for deep pleasures, but as the G-spot lies just inside the entryway to the vaginal canal, shallower thrusts will stimulate the area more directly. Shallower thrusts will also stimulate a man's glans and heighten his levels of sensitivity and arousal. Men can execute the manual methods of ejaculation control at any time during the ceremony's progression, when necessary. For example, the "squeeze method" at the base of the penis, described in the chapter "Riding the Orgasmic Wave: Male Ejaculation Control," allows the man to avoid surpassing "the point of no return," possibly even experiencing an internal orgasm, while he continues to provide the pleasures of penetration. The squeeze method also increases the fullness of the erection and permits the male partner to take a more direct and decisive aim at his target—the G-spot. If things get too hot to handle, he may opt to provide manual stimulation or use a diletto or G-spotter until he regains control.

The G-spot may also be stimulated indirectly through the fine inner membrane that separates the rectum from the vaginal canal during anal sex. Do not forget that anal-to-vaginal contact is absolutely forbidden, whether it is performed with the fingers, the penis, or any other tool. If either you or your partner have touched the anus, you must wash your hands, remove your latex gloves, or change the condom before touching the vulva or the vagina—careless anal-to-vaginal contact is almost guaranteed to result in vaginal infection. Vaginal irritation and a trip to the pharmacy should not be what women wake up to after an evening of transcendental sex!

RELAXING INTO THE PLEASURE

During G-spot stimulation, the intensity of the strokes should gradually increase, echoing the woman's levels of arousal and sensitivity. Firm pressure and more decisive strokes will soon cause distinct tingling sensations to emanate from the highly aroused G-spot. The sensations are also commonly described as flutters, pulses, or chills, and some women wrongly associate them with the need to urinate. In reality, these signals from the pelvic splanchnic nerve represent the first phase of the G-spot orgasm, as well as the first signs of imminent ejaculation. Learning to relax into the sensations of G-spot stimulation, rather than suppressing them, will open an entirely new dimension in the pleasure realm.

Women, because these signals from the pelvic splanchnic nerve are commonly misinterpreted as a pressing need to urinate, make sure to relieve yourself before beginning the Paradise Found Sexual Ceremony (and at any other time you feel the need during the course of it). Soon you will learn to recognize the difference between G-spot sensations and those that signal the need to empty your bladder.

If the G-spot is stimulated continuously, the tingling sensations emanating from it will increase in intensity. Women should breathe into these sensations and try to visualize their vibrating force. This will coax the sensations to spread down to the toes and out to the fingertips. They may even radiate straight up to the top of the head. Women, the more you are mentally present and aware of these sensations, the more sexual energy will build and flow throughout the entire body. Let your lover know just how good he or she is making you feel when you begin to sense the radiating, full-body effects of G-spot stimulation, as they are a very clear indication that your pleasure is peaking and emission is imminent.

Even though the degree of ecstatic pleasure that you begin to experience may seem unbearable, you or your partner should continue to stimulate the G-spot. When pleasure peaks, consciously prevent your PC muscle from tensing. Instead, as you do in the PC muscle flex, push the muscle gently downward and then relax the PC muscle completely. This "push and relax" technique is intrinsic to a woman's ability to ejaculate or squirt. Those who eventually unveil the powers of G-spot stimulation that lead to emission will find that this technique will become natural, if not automatic, with experience.

Developing greater PC muscle strength increases a woman's awareness of her genitals, intensifying her overall perception of the pleasures that genital stimulation provides. Flexing the PC muscles as an exercise, as described in the chapter "The Genital Gym: Strengthening the Pubococcygeal Muscle," helps to retrain the body to respond positively to ejaculation and squirting. During the heightened pleasures in the Sexual Ceremony, flexing the PC muscle will prompt the flow of ejaculate fluid into the prostate.

Most women actually cannot emit while they are being penetrated deeply or when direct pressure is applied to the G-spot. In time, you and your partner will learn to anticipate the point of emission, signaled by fluttering sensations and the complete relaxation of the vaginal walls. At first, you may need to guide your lover, either physically or verbally, but over time, he or she will learn to interpret and respond effectively to the downward push of the vaginal walls. At this time, the object of penetration should be pulled out to the very edge of the vaginal opening. If sexual tension has mounted gradually, and the orgasm (or orgasms) and all of the pleasures that lead to its exhilarating manifestation have been embraced, you and your partner are likely to witness the phenomena of female emission.

But women, if you do not experience emission, don't put pressure on yourself. Resume stroking your G-spot in the same deep, decisive manner or invite your partner to continue to stroke it, or divert your attention to other forms of stimulation and try again later. Sexual tension will continue to mount as long as you continue to play.

In the case that you and your lover succeed in opening the levee of the sacred river, revel in the liberating and, needless to say, wet sense of release and overall well-being it instills. After you have bathed in the afterglow, you will probably feel inclined to thank your lover for his or her generosity by providing some of your own undivided attention.

THE FRUITS OF THE VOYAGE

No matter what kind of stimulation is provided, as long as the woman continues to be aroused, fluid will continue to be produced within the prostate. If partners engage in the pleasures of penetration once again, they are likely to discover that the G-spot is highly sensitive to even the most subtle forms of contact, and ejaculation and squirting can now become integrated into the extended playtime of the ceremony.

As female ejaculation does not impose a refractory period, it does not slow the progression of the Sexual Ceremony, and ejaculation may occur again and again over the course of the ceremony's evolution. In that case, the time between a woman's consecutive emissions is likely to diminish, and the quantity of the liquids that each emission generates may also be augmented. These elements will also depend upon the levels of sexual skill, awareness, and acceptance as well as the degrees of arousal and desire of both partners.

After repeated and particularly abundant emissions, some women may experience the equivalent of men's "little death," the need to rest and recuperate. Others may have a sudden craving for mineral-rich foods. (I personally crave oysters and anchovies!) Women, allow your body to be your guide; take an intermission in the Sexual Ceremony if you feel the need, and, throughout the ceremony, remember to drink plenty of mineral water. Female squirting can result in the loss of a lot of precious fluid.

During intense periods of ecstatic stimulation and repeated ejaculation or squirting, women are likely to experience unprecedented degrees of genital swelling and sensitivity. Lovers, on that occasion, use a handheld mirror to get a view of the genitals and share in the vision. Plump with love, all of the visible elements of the clitoral system will be engorged and highly receptive to touch. The tissues surrounding the urethra may even swell to dimensions comparable in size to the clitoris. When the G-spot and the U-spot are thus engorged with excitement and highly sensitized, they may be stimulated orally to ecstatic effect, provoking U-spot and G-spot orgasms, as well as emission.

Repeated ejaculation, in combination with multiple orgasms—whether they occur in association with each other or separately as a response to heightened degrees of pleasure—will provoke a surge of endorphins into the bloodstream and incite a sexual high. Over long periods of arousal, an uninterrupted free flow of sexual energy may also be induced, which has been described as an extended or massive orgasm. This is what men experience when they learn to ride the waves of climax over and over again during long periods of arousal.

Instigating the buildup of emissions takes time, skill, and loving attention, and some women may simply need more time to awaken their G-spot than others. And not everyone can shed the negative repercussions that the pleasure taboo has heaped upon bodies, minds, and spirits over the past two thousand years. However, partners who refrain from creating performance anxiety and regularly practice direct G-spot stimulation are likely to experience the prostatic flux sooner or later.

Also with practice, partners will discover the sexual positions that are most favorable to G-spot orgasms and emission. Some women may prefer to be on top of male partners, while others will respond when they are penetrated from behind. Some like reclining in a sling—a form of hammock designed to either hang from the ceiling or from a four-post structure—or sitting on a high countertop that puts their genitals at the height of their partner's object of penetration, be it a penis, finger, or diletto. This position allows both partners to see everything—from her (and his) swollen sex to her jets of ecstasy. There are no rules—experiment, enjoy the journey, and transcend together!

CHAPTER 6

o

THE ANTHEMS OF ANAL SEX: FROM HYGIENE TO HEAVENLY PLEASURES

Out beyond ideas of wrongdoing and right doing, there is a field.
I will meet you there . . .

— Rumi

EXPLORING THE long-forbidden frontier of the anus and learning to enjoy anal stimulation are not essential to the Paradise Found Sexual Ceremony, but I encourage all lovers, whatever their sexual orientation, to set aside anal taboos. The anus, composed of erectile tissues that are charged with nerve endings, has the potential to provide unique, ecstatic sensations, and it goes without saying that the organ's proximity to the genitals also renders it impossible to ignore! After all, the anus is a part of our anatomy, and anal stimulation—whether it leads to penetration or not—can be considered another option in the vast repertoire of pleasures that lovers may enjoy during the Sexual Ceremony.

Part of the goal of this chapter is to dismantle the taboos that surround the "rosebud" (as it is affectionately called by the British)—taboos that inhibit many from partaking in the ecstatic joys of anal stimulation. Because many lovers avoid the anus for fear of encountering feces, this chapter also explores methods of anal hygiene in preparation for the pleasures that lie ahead on our sexual horizons.

Because the anus is a source of shame and inhibition for many, verbal or physical consent is crucial before attempting to give or receive any form of anal stimulation, even between partners who are normally receptive to such pleasures. As needs and desires change from day to day, what gives someone bliss one day might not be the case the next.

FROM ACCEPTANCE TO CONDEMNATION

The sexual preferences and behaviors of pre-Abrahamic cultures were influenced less by questions of morality than by freely chosen personal tastes. The Greeks and Romans did not consider the anus a taboo area, nor did they associate anally derived pleasures solely with homosexuality. However shocking it may be to us today, pederasty between a teacher and his students was seen as a means to impart wisdom. In his *The History of Sexuality*, a three-volume work published between 1976 and 1984, the philosopher Michel Foucault explains that there were no homosexuals in the ancient world, only homosexual acts and practices. What we call bisexuality today was considered to be a normal expression of sexuality—a natural, erotic response to truth, beauty, and virtue. Homosexual acts between sexually mature adults, male or female, were tolerated, if not accepted, although those who engaged exclusively in same-sex relations were viewed under slightly less favorable terms. The most blatant exception to this rule can be found in Plato's *The Symposium*. Plato argued that armies should ideally be composed of same-sex lovers. The Sacred Band of Thebes was formed with three hundred male soldiers who met this prerequisite; they were renowned in the ancient world for their dauntless courage in battle. I like to believe that it was the invaluable sentiment of love and their vital desire to continue loving that led these men to be such heroic fighters!

The decline of the Roman Empire saw the rise of Christianity, marking the fall of the Western world's freedom of sexual expression. By 500 A.D., sodomy had become synonymous with sin, as did same-sex relations and any other sexual behavior enjoyed purely for the sake of pleasure and not for procreation. Of course, this did not put an end to sex for the sake of sex, but it became the foundation for the pleasure taboo.

The term "homosexual," relating to the homosexual identity as we understand it today, did not emerge until the end of the nineteenth century. It is attributed to British physician, psychologist, and social reformer Havelock Ellis, the author of *Sexual Inversion*. Written in 1896, this was the first medical textbook to deal objectively with homosexuality.

Austrian psychoanalyst Sigmund Freud was the first sexual researcher to take an openly positive stance in regard to anal eroticism, but his conclusions were limited to childhood development. He concluded that children instinctively procure auto-gratification via the erogenous zones of the body in three stages—beginning with the mouth at birth (the oral stage), the anus at approximately one and a half years (the anal stage), and finally the genitals, at approximately three years (the phallic stage).

According to Freud, during the anal stages of infantile sexuality, both anal sensations and anal functions (the expulsion or retention of feces) become a child's psychosexual obsession. Freud declared the pleasures thus derived to be natural, even fundamental, aspects of childhood development. He reduced the derivation of anally derived pleasure in sexually mature adults, on the other hand, to childish behavior—the consequence of developmental arrest during the anal stage of development.

Freud openly declared that same-sex attraction between humans is natural, and that bisexuality is innate, but like his contemporaries, he failed to more profoundly address, much less advocate, the equally controversial topic of anal eroticism in adults. To do so at the turn of the twentieth century would undoubtedly have posed a certain risk, considering that sodomy was still deemed to be abnormal and even pathological. Anyone who engaged in such pleasures, male or female, was at peril of being persecuted, put under medical treatment, or both. Freud's failure to address the topic of anal pleasure in sexually mature adults may have also been defensive. His homosexual inclinations, in particular toward his disciples Sándor Ferenczi and Carl Jung, are not the best-kept secrets.

It was not until the sexual liberation movement went into full swing at the end of the 1960s that sociosexual mores would begin to change. But certain behaviors remain controversial, including sodomy and same-sex relations. In spite of Gay Pride, which was jump-started by the Stonewall riots on June 29, 1969, in New York City, persecution of homosexuals is still promulgated in the medical and psychiatric spheres, and clinics that claim to "cure" homosexuality still exist. Due in part to the fact that information concerning anal health and pleasure is still mostly confined to the male homosexual community, the myths and misconceptions surrounding the topic of anal sex have yet to be completely debunked.

While heterosexual men may be reluctant to receive anal stimulation, they have been traditionally much less hesitant about providing it for their female partners. There is probably not a single culture that has not recognized anal sex as the most obvious way to partake in the pleasures of penetration with women without paying the procreative consequences. (In reality, anal sex is not 100 percent effective as a form of birth control. If semen leaks out of the anus, eager sperm may also swim into the Fallopian tubes via the crimson warmth of the uterus, where their sole mission in life may be accomplished—union with a ready ovum.)

ANAL TABOOS: ALLEVIATING ANAL ANXIETIES

Most straight men are reluctant to engage in anal stimulation, believing that if they accept and enjoy anal contact, their female partner will accuse them of "being gay," or that they will "turn" homosexual. But it should be understood that this pleasure is *not* the sole provenance of the homosexual male! Charged with nerve endings, the anus is capable of providing intensely pleasant sensations. Penetrating the anus also happens to be the only direct way to access a man's prostate gland or P-spot (the anatomical equivalent of the female G-spot) and revel in the deep, full-body sensations that manual stimulation can provide.

Before the discovery of the female prostate, the anus was considered to be the only part of the sexual anatomy that both men and women had, and therefore the only source of sexual pleasure that might be physically compared. As with the idea of female ejaculation, disconcerting gender similarities may be one subtle reason that anal sex became, and remains deeply rooted in, taboo.

The functions of the rectum and anus to retain and eliminate waste is the least subtle reason why many consider these bodily parts with repulsion and shame. This primal aversion is ingrained in each of us; even the most sexually liberated of parents will unthinkingly transmit the anal taboo to their children. The slightest grimace of disgust, repeated during diaper change after diaper change, day after day for at least two years of every child's life, is bound to make an impact on the way that child feels about the anus and its function by the time he or she reaches adulthood. (Parents, make a conscious effort to smile at your babies during diaper changes, and you will make a proactive gesture toward dismantling the anal taboo in subsequent generations.)

Another fear that inhibits lovers from engaging in anal sex, no matter their gender or sexual orientation, is that the practice will inevitably entail pain. It's true that the sensitive anus can be a source of extreme agony when mistreated. But when it is approached with care, skill, and consent, the anus can provide equally extreme degrees of pleasure! Extended playtime and heightened states of arousal will cause the anus to swell and dilate, just like the genitals, rendering it receptive to stimulation. Having something enter or exit your anus is easier upon your exhalation, so it is important to remember to breathe! If you are the one providing the pleasure, let your partner's breath be your guide. Because the anus does not self-lubricate like the vagina, the abundant use of lubricants is essential to pleasurable anal stimulation.

LUBRICANTS—THE ANAL STIMULATION IMPERATIVE

Silicone-, glycerin-, or water-based lubricants eliminate the friction that we associate with discomfort. It also eliminates the chafing and irritation that may be experienced with the use of latex condoms, with the added advantage of minimizing condom breakage. While saliva will do in a pinch if a partner is highly aroused, receptive, and therefore dilated, it is not as effective as lubricants designed specifically for enhanced sexual pleasure.

Oil-based lubricants such as olive oil or the baking ingredient Crisco (a hydrogenated oil) are not safe alternatives to lubrication. As conducive as they may be to penetration, they leave insoluble residues in the anal (or vaginal) canal that are difficult for the body to eliminate. And oils are *not* latex friendly! This includes "baby oil"—a common bedside component. The use of oils in the boudoir should be reserved for the purpose of massaging the body, not the genitals or the anus.

ANAL ANATOMY

The digestive tract begins with the mouth and ends with the anus. It includes the esophagus, stomach, small and large intestines, rectum, and anal canal, sometimes called the lower rectum. Two muscles, the internal and the external anal sphincters, surround the margin of the anus. Our ability to consciously relax the external sphincter muscles, which are composed of skeletal, or striated, muscle and so lie under our voluntary control, is essential to regulating the pleasures of anal penetration. The internal anal sphincter, composed of smooth muscle, is an involuntary muscle that works in tandem with the external sphincter and can therefore also be coaxed to cooperate.

The best example of the difference between internal and external anal sphincter control manifests itself when the brain receives the impulse to evacuate. The internal anal sphincter reflexively holds back the fecal material. Under normal conditions, we go immediately to the toilet; but if that release is not readily available, we are obliged to hold it by tightening the external sphincter muscles until we can find relief. Those who practice the genital gym, described in the chapter "The Genital Gym: Strengthening the Pubococcygeal Muscle," will develop greater sphincter muscle awareness and control, which is crucial to the pleasures of anal penetration.

HAIL THE BARRIERS!

Before proceeding, it's important to mention the potential but avoidable hazards of anal sex. When anal stimulation or penetration is practiced without barriers, it becomes the highest-risk form of intimate contact. The tissues of the anus, anal canal, and rectum are as capable of transmitting and contracting venereal disease as the vagina, and unsafe anal penetration remains the most common means of HIV transmission. The delicate tissues of that area are extremely fragile, increasing the likelihood of encountering blood, the most efficient carrier of the HIV virus. Lovers who are not bound by an exclusive and safe fluid-exchange agreement must protect themselves with a barrier at all times.

Barriers serve not only to prevent the transmission of STDs but also to provide a sensation of cleanliness. Those who are fearful of encountering feces will feel more at ease when barriers are used, and therefore more receptive to pleasure. In addition, fecal matter, only considered erotic by scatophiles, is potentially dangerous; even healthy feces can contain toxins and bacteria.

Condoms, dental dams, and latex gloves are a must if anal pleasures are part of the ceremonial plan. And be prepared: make sure your barriers are close at hand before the Paradise Found Sexual Ceremony begins.

Uninhibited aficionados of anal sex are likely to enjoy the pleasures of anilingus, also called "rimming." Unless a thorough anal cleansing has been done and partners have a safe fluid-exchange agreement, those who enjoy oral-to-anal contact should always protect each other with barriers. Anilingus presents exactly the same risks as oral-to-genital contact, and the best way to avoid these risks is through the use of dental dams. These thin sheets of latex can be stretched over the anus to keep the tongue, lips, and mouth from contacting germs and fecal matter. Ordinarily used by dentists to isolate a tooth or teeth from the rest of the oral cavity, dental dams may be purchased on the Internet, in some sex shops, and in any dental supply store.

If you don't have a dam, and you are uncertain that the person you are "consuming" is disease free, a sheet of plastic wrap (yes, the kind that preserves food) can be used as an equally effective means of preserving your health and the health of your partner. A condom can also be used. To create a dam from a condom, cut off its tip with a pair of sharp scissors. Then cut the resulting tube in half. This will create a latex sheet that will allow you to engage in safe rimming. Condoms designed specifically for women have a wide brim and may also be used for anal play. Unfortunately, these condoms are not as easy to find as they should be.

To create a dam from a latex glove, first cut away the four fingers, then cut the glove in half, straight down the side and opposite the thumb, which should be left intact (leave enough material to provide sufficient coverage). The result is a sheet of latex with an attached, closed funnel, which can be used to anchor the dam inside the anus. The "glove dam" will allow you to penetrate orally with greater ease than a flat barrier and with less risk. But don't forget: if the glove contains talc, before using it as a dam, rinse it with warm, soapy water and pat dry.

Before using any oral barrier, mark the side that will *not* come into contact with the body with a waterproof pen. Otherwise your good intentions to "play safe" are all for naught! Also apply a thin layer of lubrication to the anal area, which will cause the barrier to adhere to the skin. If using a "glove dam," apply abundant lubrication to the closed funnel shape as well before inserting it into the anus.

During manual stimulation or penetration of the anus, I highly recommend that you wear talc-free latex gloves. They prevent the delicate tissues of the receiver's anus from being unintentionally damaged by a fingernail and protect the provider from bacterial infection. Keep in mind that even minor scratches or micro-abrasions on the hands may allow germs to enter the body. No matter how small anal injuries may be, their healing is a long and uncomfortable process. Needless to say, any form of anal contact should be avoided in the presence of wounds; the healing process would be aggravated by the stimulations of sexual activity.

INSTRUMENTS FOR BLISSFUL ANAL PLAY

Plugs, prostate stimulators, vibrators, beads, and dilettos that are designed specifically for anal penetration either have a graduated or flared end or they are long enough to hold a generous portion of the total length firmly in hand. This prevents them from slipping into the rectum or beyond, and thereby guarantee that you won't find yourself in the emergency room!

If your partner is female, consider providing her with double the pleasure, letting her experience an unequivocal sense of fullness through the simultaneous penetration of both the anus and the vagina with the help of a diletto. The G-spot will receive a delightful degree of pressure that will flood the female prostate with ejaculate fluid.

If you are inserting into the anus any object other than fingers, a penis, or a strap-on diletto that has an ergonomic form, proceed with care and patience. Remember that the walls of the rectum require time to conform to the inserted object. If your lover is feeling anything but pleasure and emotional bliss, slow down. *Never* fail to respect your partner's wishes if he or she asks you to exit altogether.

CLEANLINESS BEGINS FROM WITHIN

While the use of barriers will reduce tensions and inhibitions that many lovers associate with anal stimulation, the only way to completely extinguish the fear of encountering feces is to eliminate them from the rectum altogether. Making simple cleansing preparations before the Sexual Ceremony will facilitate your own and your lover's comfort and sense of security.

Anal cleanliness begins from within. The way in which we nourish ourselves determines not only how we look and feel but how our digestive tract functions, too. The more balanced our diets are, the cleaner the entire organism will be. A high-fiber diet makes for more solid excrement, which is easier for the body to eliminate and less likely to leave traces in the digestive tract. This kind of feces is a sign of intestinal health and nutritional balance. Soft feces are often a result of an unbalanced, low-fiber diet and can generate serious health problems over time. Their presence in the intestine is often accompanied with a sense of bloating, which may reduce our libido. A well-balanced, high-fiber diet should thus be considered essential to both general and sexual health.

The last organ to hold fecal material after its passage through the colon is the rectum. In your preparation for the Paradise Found Sexual Ceremony, douching will cleanse this area as well as the lower rectum (also termed the anal canal) and the anus. If it is performed an hour or so before the ceremony commences, it will stimulate bowel movement, thereby completely emptying the large intestine—a liberating feeling that is also conducive to the libido. Regardless of whether or not partners intend to engage in anal stimulation, this form of hygiene provides an overall sense of cleanliness and well-being, which always promotes sexual satisfaction.

Note that anal douching is not the same as deep colon cleansing, a.k.a. hydrocolonic cleansing or colonic irrigation. Deep colon cleansing, a treat for the body, is the work of a specialist and entails having large quantities of lukewarm water filtered through the rectum into the sigmoid colon, the S-shaped curve of the large intestine that lies closest to the rectum, and possibly farther, and then extracted again. As recovery from this cleansing and the reacclimatizing of the digestive system can take a few days, I recommend it as a longer-term treatment before the Sexual Ceremony—a gift to yourself during the change of seasons, for example, as it hydrates the entire body, eliminates toxins, and generates a healthy glow.

Mae West's Beauty Secret
Compared to deep colon cleansing, anal douching involves filtering only small quantities of water through the anus into the rectum, so it can be performed in the comfort of your own bathroom. A rectal douche is within the realm of possibility in a daily health regimen—actress Mae West declared that anal douching, which

she integrated into her daily beauty routine, was the secret behind her impeccable complexion. Another health benefit that anal douching rewards us with is relief from the symptoms of anal tension, including constipation.

As one of the most sensitive areas of the body, the anus, like the stomach and the intestines, is extremely susceptible to the repercussions of stress and negative energy. Anal tension is a common side effect of anxiety; it can cause intestinal irritation as well as constipation, leading to any number of conditions, including hemorrhoids. These conditions decrease the libido and, thus, anal receptivity. The more relaxed and healthy we feel in general, the more likely we are to be receptive to any form of sexual stimulation.

Enema bulbs and "pears" are the most common douching devices; vaginal pears can also be used anally. However, do not use the same device to administer both anal and vaginal douches. Note that vaginal douching disturbs the natural pH balance of the vagina, increasing the likelihood of infections. Unlike rectal douching, it should only be practiced under the recommendation of a doctor to treat specific medical conditions.

Enema bags, which usually hold one quart of liquid, are not only more time-consuming to use but increase the likelihood that water will fill the rectum and seep into the sigmoid colon. Being that it will take the body longer to eliminate the excess water, the use of enema bags is therefore not recommended prior to the Sexual Ceremony.

Water is the ideal solution for anal douching. Commercial douching solutions and enemas contain chemicals and so should be avoided; the chemicals will be absorbed into your system, altering the pH of the intestinal tract and its natural functions. If you purchase traditional enema bulbs containing douche solutions, empty their contents and refill them with clean, warm water.

The ideal water temperature for rectal douching is that of your body temperature, 98.6°F (37°C). Water that is too cold will cause cramping, and water that is too hot can damage the delicate tissues. Run the water over your inner wrist to ensure that it is as close to body temperature as possible before filling your douching device.

Ready, Steady, Breathe

When you're ready to give yourself a douche, follow these directions: Fill your douching device with no more than about one cup of water. (More may result in water entering the sigmoid colon and stimulating the peristaltic action of the entire intestine.) Lubricate both the nozzle of the enema bulb and your anus. Spread a towel on the bathroom floor, lie down on your left side, which eases pressure on the lower digestive tract, and make yourself comfortable. Remember that having something enter or exit your anus is easier upon your exhalation, so when you are ready, breathe out while inserting the nozzle into your anus. Relax into the sensations that penetrating the organ generates, then gradually fill the rectum with water. Your body will tell you when you reach rectal capacity by stimulating peristalsis—the evacuation reflex. Thereupon, go immediately to the toilet.

During the first cleansing you will probably also release feces that were lingering in the rectum. Resume your relaxed, supine position and repeat the process. It may take another douche or two to complete the entire elimination. Depending on how you feel, you may stop at any time. Once every trace of fecal matter held in the rectum has exited the body, the water you pass will look clear. Always wait about thirty to sixty minutes after douching before you engage in anal play, in order to be certain that all of the liquid has been eliminated from your system.

Rinse and Repeat

An easy, effective, and time-efficient alternative to traditional douching devices like pears and bulbs is the shower douche, a device designed to screw directly onto the end of a flexible shower hose, in place of the showerhead. It normally has a tubular-shaped nozzle, but it may also take the form of an anal plug. Shower douches are available today through most male-oriented sex shops, as well as online, but equally effective results may be attained through the following procedure, if you have a showerhead attached to a flexible hose.

First unscrew the showerhead. If the attachment has a loose rubber seal, set that aside in order to avoid its slipping down the drain. Adjust the temperature of the water and its pressure so that it exits the hose at the slowest jet possible. While sitting on the edge of the bathtub, or assuming a squatting position in the shower, position the end of the hose against—*not inside*—the anal orifice. Allow the water to gradually fill the anal canal and rectum. This will take only a few seconds. Exercise control over your sphincter muscles, and go straight to the toilet. Repeat the process, until clear water exits the body.

If you suffer from anal anxiety, you may not wish to do any form of anal douching, even though it is the most effective way to ensure cleanliness; however, no one should feel obliged to undergo the procedure. Fecal particles can, in fact, also be removed manually while you are bathing or showering. Manual cleansing also provides an excellent opportunity to develop a greater sense of anal awareness and acceptance. Take care to avoid letting soap enter the anal canal, as it is likely to irritate the tissues of the rectum. Establish a deep, regular breathing pattern to relax mind and body; upon exhalation, penetrate the anus with your middle finger; and remove any stagnant fecal matter. You may find there is actually very little residue in the anal canal if you are eating a high-fiber diet and your feces are solid. For optimal hygiene and to keep fingernails from injuring tender tissues, use latex gloves.

Being that excrement moves continuously through the small

intestine into the colon and the rectum, anal cleansing, no matter the method you prefer, can be repeated during intermissions of lengthy sexual rituals, if and when the need arises.

ROSEBUD PLAY

Once the "rosebud" has been cleansed, it can be approached with peace of mind. Novices to the pleasures of anal stimulation may learn to explore the anus in the solo masturbation ritual before incorporating anal play into the Paradise Found Sexual Ceremony, and I hope that you find that bonding with this part of your sexual anatomy is more pleasurable than you ever imagined!

Use a handheld mirror to look at your anus while exploring its outer area manually. Use plenty of lubrication and take your time. When you feel ready, proceed inward to discover the anal canal and the soft walls of the rectum. The anus itself represents the greatest concentration of nerve endings in the anal area, so keep in mind that the rectum, like the vagina, is more sensitive in its first third of depth, as measured from the collar of the anus. Become aware of all of the sensations that stimulating and penetrating the orifice provides. As you learn to accept the sensitive organ as an ally in pleasure, the anxieties you may have associated with it will gradually dissolve.

The following guidance to anal play is from the point of view of the *provider* of such pleasures; if your erotic desire is to be on the *receiving* end, these instructions will provide insight into how you can direct your lover. If you are disinclined to explore anal play, please don't skip over this section! Reading through it will help you to understand why others desire such pleasures—and it is through this kind of understanding that we evolve further along our own sexual paths.

If you are playing with a partner who is normally receptive to anal stimulation, remember that it is still important to obtain his or her consent before engaging in anal play. If you know your lover well enough to read his or her body language, this can be as simple as gently testing your partner's receptivity. Otherwise, ask for permission. If your partner is in the mood, apply lubricant and take the time to tantalize and entice the anus to reception with the tips of your fingers, your tongue, or your lips. If your intention is to penetrate your lover's anus, these pleasures must be considered essential preliminaries.

Invitation to Advance

Once your consenting lover is genuinely relaxed and aroused, and his or her anus has swollen to receptive excitement, you may attempt to advance inward. Before proceeding to do so, abundant lubrication should be reapplied externally and, ideally, internally, too. This is possible through the use of lubrication syringes, which may be purchased in male-oriented sex shops or on the Internet. Traditional syringes will also work equally well. Once you have removed and properly disposed of the needle, fill the syringe with lubricant.

Ask your aroused lover to take a deep breath and hold it for a few seconds before exhaling. Upon his or her exhalation, slowly insert the tip of the syringe into the anus and inject the lubricant. Set the syringe aside nearby, as you may need to make consecutive applications as the ritual proceeds. Anal penetration should always be slow-going, while communication should always be free-flowing.

You can now stimulate the entryway to the anal canal. If your lover is a novice, invite him or her to take a deep breath, and upon the exhalation, penetrate his or her anus by applying light pressure to its center with the tip of the middle finger. The middle finger is an ideal tool for the initial phases of penetration (some lovers consider it to be the only tool!). Those who enjoy being penetrated with more than one finger, or with a penis or dilettos, will still usually need to be dilated with a smaller object first. The middle finger serves this purpose well.

Once inside, gradually enter the orifice up to approximately the first knuckle of your middle finger—then *don't move*. Stay still, and allow your lover to ease into the sensations and control the depth of penetration. You will soon feel his or her anal sphincters begin to relax. If you sense that your partner is tense, invite him or her to breathe deeply—filling lungs to capacity, holding the breath briefly at the end of the inhalation, and exhaling slowly while consciously relaxing all of the muscles that compose the genital system, including the sphincters—to facilitate penetration. This manner of breathing will also heighten your partner's perception of pleasure.

As anal tension subsides, continue to massage the walls of the anal canal slowly and patiently. Stroke its muscular walls in circular patterns, but patiently refrain from advancing inward. (Remember that no one is obliged to accept penetration, but if your lover is enjoying what you are doing, he or she is likely to beg you to proceed!)

Grant Your Lover's Wishes

Once you feel the walls relax, you may begin to move gradually inward. Be aware of his or her breathing pattern at all times. If your lover forgets to breathe regularly, remind him or her to do so. Continue massaging the muscular anal canal in circular patterns while working inward gradually and lovingly.

If at any moment your lover seems to be experiencing anything but pleasure and emotional bliss, slow down. If your lover doesn't ease into the sensations, ask what you can do to make him or her more comfortable. If you are asked to stop what you are doing, respect those wishes, and, first inviting your lover to breathe in deeply, exit his or her body upon exhalation as carefully and patiently as you entered.

If, on the other hand, your lover is enjoying the exploration, you may continue on. You will notice that as arousal grows, the sphincter muscles will grow noticeably more supple and receptive, and you will be able to pass into the anal canal and outward again with ease. Allow your lover to guide you both physically and verbally at all times. In preparation for deeper penetration, lubrication can be reapplied if necessary. This time, you will be able to insert the syringe deeper into the anal canal; slowly inject its entire contents directly into the rectum. Remove the syringe on your lover's exhalation and proceed to re-penetrate the anus, granting your lover's wishes.

Once you have penetrated the entire length of the anal canal, you may have the opportunity to explore the soft walls of the rectum, as long as your lover is receptive. Make a mental note of its shape and its sweet curve. Your understanding of its particularities will be important if you plan to engage in more advanced play, especially if it involves the use of dilettos, which may not correspond exactly to its curve. Always make sure that the anus is well dilated before inserting a diletto, penis, or more than one finger.

Note that when the genitals are stimulated during anal penetration, by either of you, the anal sphincters will clamp firmly down around your finger (or other object of penetration). This reaction should not be confused with anal tension. On the contrary, as soon as genital stimulation ceases, you will notice that the sphincters will relax even more, ready to reacquaint themselves with more delightful intrusions.

If your partner is male, his penis may not necessarily become erect during anal penetration, which is not indicative of the degree of pleasure that he is experiencing. Some men simply prefer to revel in one pleasure or the other—the simultaneous provision of anal penetration and genital stimulation can cause sensory overload and distract him from enjoying either pleasure to the fullest.

Whether you are male or female, indulging in the delectable joys of skillful anal penetration can incite unprecedented states of heightened sexual arousal. By setting shame and inhibition aside, we can reap more of the titillating benefits that sexual bliss bestow upon body, mind, and spirit.

TARGETING THE DIVINE P-SPOT

The anus provides access to the divine P-spot in men, but if your lover is a woman and thoroughly enjoys anal penetration, once you have dilated her anus enough to penetrate it comfortably, you may use your penis or diletto to target her G-spot through the wall that divides the vaginal canal from the anal canal. Remember that careless anal-to-vaginal contact is likely to cause infection.

If your partner is male and is thoroughly enjoying himself, once the muscular anal canal has been surpassed, you may locate the prostate gland. It lies approximately 3 inches (7 centimeters) inside the anal canal, behind the upper wall of the rectum. It can be found by making a "come hither" gesture with your inserted finger, in the direction of the navel. The prostate gland is often referred to as the "P-spot" to reinforce its similarities with the female G-spot, and, like the female prostate, the male prostate tends to respond better to deep, circular strokes and firm, controlled pressure. Once you have made contact with the organ, take your time to gradually and carefully explore its shape, size, and texture. These characteristics will vary slightly from male to male, but a healthy prostate normally presents itself in a smooth, firm state, with well-rounded contours and a slightly indented center.

With care and erotic intent, proceed to gently massage the prostate along its outer edges, rather than in its center (unless your lover tells you to do otherwise). Its distinctive, ovoid chestnut shape will have become swollen with pleasure. The more a man is aroused, the more blood will rush toward the P-spot, rendering the gland increasingly sensitive. Heightened degrees of arousal also incite the production of ejaculate fluid. While every prostate differs slightly in size and consistency, they all share the same capacity to bestow deeply satisfying sensations.

During prostate stimulation, remain aware of your lover's responses, and regulate the depth and intensity of the massage accordingly. As long as the receiver is ecstatically reveling, direct contact may continue. Again, let your lover be your guide, verbally and physically, at all times.

As his excitement mounts, you may feel the organ pulsing under your fingertip; this is known as the "prostate flutter." If the man practices a consciously controlled breathing pattern, the energy now being generated inside the gland may be coaxed to spread throughout the entire body. P-spot stimulation is hailed for sparking deep, full-body pleasure. Some men claim the intensity of the sensations of direct contact with the prostate to be equal, if not superior, to those created by genital stimulation.

During heightened degrees of arousal, men may emit prostate fluid with the P-spot orgasm. Like semen, this fluid is white in color, but its consistency is denser than semen; it actually lends the male emission its distinctive characteristics. P-spot orgasms that result in prostate-fluid emission do not emit sperm and so do not compromise the erection or, therefore, the progression of the Sexual Ceremony.

Prostate massage invites fresh, oxygenated blood to circulate through the gland; it provides sexual pleasure and also keeps the organ toned. While one man learns to appreciate anal penetration and prostate massage, another will remain adamant about not having his anus penetrated, much less his prostate stimulated. But sooner or later, virtually every man will become familiar with his prostate—at the doctor's office! Prostate problems usually manifest in men over sixty years of age. Could this be due to a lack of prostate stimulation?

If you do not wish to allow your partner to stimulate your prostate gland, you might consider doing so, on your own, during masturbation. This should ideally be done in coordination with exercises detailed in the chapter "The Genital Gym: Strengthening the Pubococcygeal Muscle" in order to heighten your anal awareness and bring fresh, oxygenated blood to the area. This will gradually reduce anal tension and facilitate penetration.

Men, if you are not comfortable with penetration, the prostate can also be located and massaged externally during masturbation, via the perineum, with your fingers or knuckles. During the exercise, the entirety of the lower penile shaft, which extends from the base of the scrotum and down toward the anus, should also be massaged with slow, firm gestures.

When you are well aroused, locate the indentation that lies in the area just below the anus. Firmly press the perineal wall inward and upward until you feel distinct, pulsating sensations emanating from the prostate, then gradually apply deeper pressure to the gland. Folding the knees toward the chest will facilitate access to this portion of the perineum and permit for a deeper massage. Some men find that the area of the perineum that lies closer to the scrotum also provides similar sensations. Explore, and you will discover what works best for you. While the effects of the external stimulation are not as immediate as when the prostate is approached internally, they will provide pleasure all the same. And becoming familiar with and learning to accept this aspect of your sexual anatomy may eventually tempt you to discover the enhanced sensations of prostate massage through anal play.

EASY ACCESS

The ideal position to facilitate anal stimulation and penetration, as well as prostate massage, will differ from person to person. You might like to lie on your back with legs extended and knees bent up toward the chest as described above, or with the feet planted firmly on the surface on which you are lying. The latter position allows you to have greater control over the movement of your hips and, therefore the depth of penetration. You might prefer to position your buttocks on the edge of a bed for the same reasons, as well as to facilitate entry. If you are a novice to anal penetration, you might prefer lying on your back, which has the added advantage of permitting direct eye contact with the provider of your pleasure, and thus both verbal and nonverbal communication. If you are more experienced, you might enjoy being penetrated while bound (see plate VI, page 118) or from behind—either while lying flat on your stomach, bending forward and bracing yourself from a standing position, or positioning yourself on all fours.

The anal-penetration aficionado often invests in a sling. This type of hammock is sometimes reinforced to be more flat and rigid. Slings provide numerous advantages beyond easy anal access; most enticingly, because the body is suspended in air, slings induce an immediate feeling of floating relaxation that lends itself to receptivity.

Experimentation will reveal the positions that work best for each individual. No matter the details, anal penetration should always be performed gradually and in harmony with the receiving partner's needs and desires. However small or large the favored object of penetration may be, if the receiver is fully aroused and relaxed, you will note with delight how his or her sphincter will cease resisting penetration and actually begin to suck the penetrator inward. The depth of the thrusts should then be regulated according to the lover's needs and desires.

The anal arena should be a source of exhilarating and intensely gratifying pleasure, for both women and men, no matter their sexual orientation. Embrace the anus and the interrelated internal organs as integrated parts of their sexual anatomy, and expand your sexual repertoire!

PARADISE FOUND: THE SEXUAL CEREMONY

In which Paradise beckons, and lovers abandon themselves to the profound sensual pleasures that rule the realm of erotic revelry.

THE ANCIENT GREEKS planned and carried out elaborate sexual rituals, both privately and publicly, in the form of the sacred orgy. As well as providing the attainment of deep satisfaction, sex was a spiritual endeavor—a means of venerating the gods and goddesses. On days of worship, temples dedicated to Aphrodite, the goddess of love and beauty, Demeter, the goddess of fertility, and Dionysus, the god of wine and ecstasy, were purified and decorated with the intent to cater to the senses, promote erotic revelry, and coax devotees to abandon themselves to the sexual realm.

Bathing was an important aspect of their sexual ceremonies; water, like food and wine, was plentiful. The aroma of incense and fresh flowers mingled with the distinct musk of sex and rose to the heavens. Soft cushions made of finely woven fabrics from faraway lands framed the libidinous landscape of inebriated lovers gyrating in harmony to lascivious tunes wafting from the flutes and lyres of dancing *auletrides*. These sultry sacred prostitutes helped the hetaerae—the most seductive, powerful, and wealthy women in ancient Greece—to fund, with the art of loving, the raising of some of the most lavish temples in the ancient world.

The goal of the devoted worshippers was to become one with themselves, their partners, and ultimately with the gods and goddesses who commanded the generating forces of the universe. Body, mind, and spirit became charged with the sexual vibration over the course of extended periods of arousal as lovers merged.

Such sacred rituals are an ecstatic source of inspiration for your elaboration of the Paradise Found Sexual Ceremony—whether you are married or single, heterosexual or homosexual, have children or not. By learning to engage the entire body, mind, and spirit as a sexual, sensual whole, lovers transcend the doldrums of predominantly genitally oriented (PGO) sex to experience together the greater dimensions of the sacred realm of pleasure.

This transcension evolves spontaneously, ritual after creative ritual, when lovers are emotionally connected and experienced in the arts of the Sexual Ceremony. But if an experienced lover wishes to initiate a novice and share its powers, this should be done gradually and only with his or her consent.

The Sexual Ceremony begins with mindful preparation, which transforms into sexual anticipation; continues in the development and evolution of sexual pleasures with a partner, transforming the

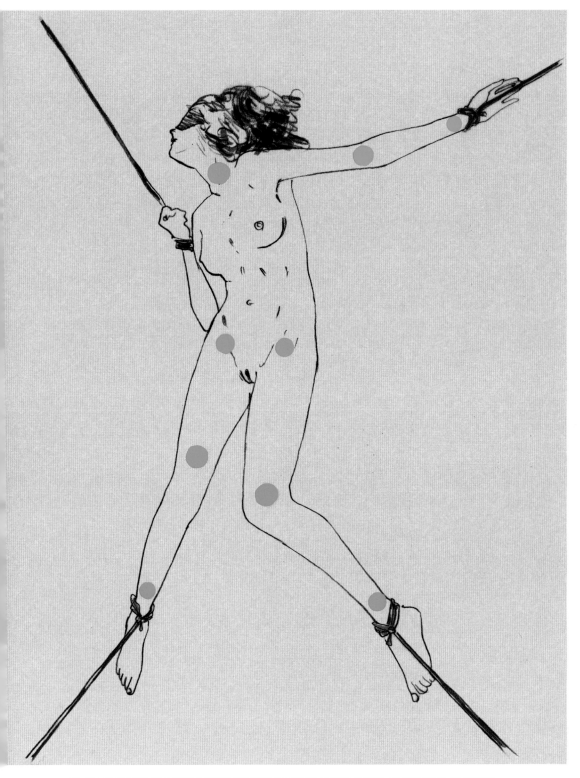

PLATE IX BONDAGE SESSION WITH FRENCH BOWLINE (CORD CUFFS), SHOWING "NO" ZONES

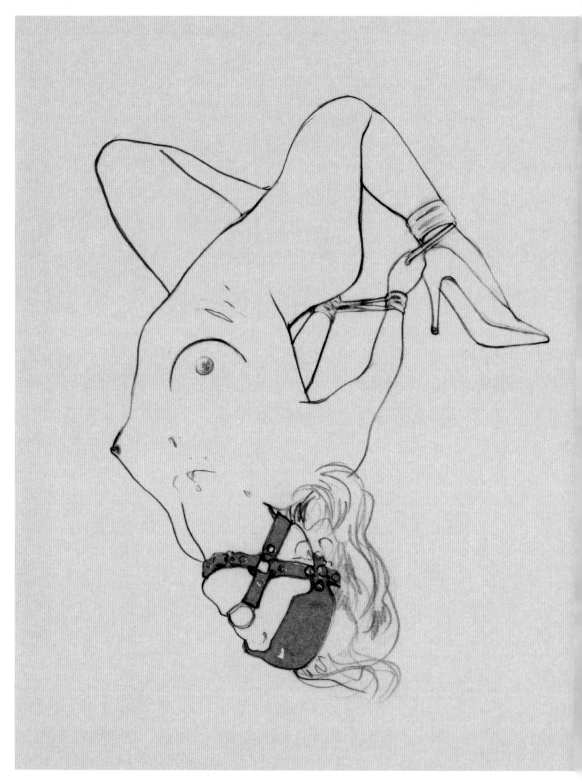

PLATE X BONDAGE SESSION WITH BLINDFOLD AND MOUTH GAG

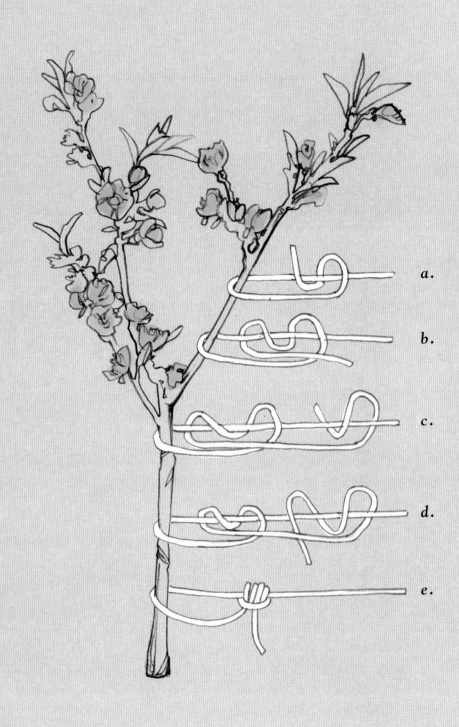

a.

b.

c.

d.

e.

PLATE XI THE PRUSIK KNOT

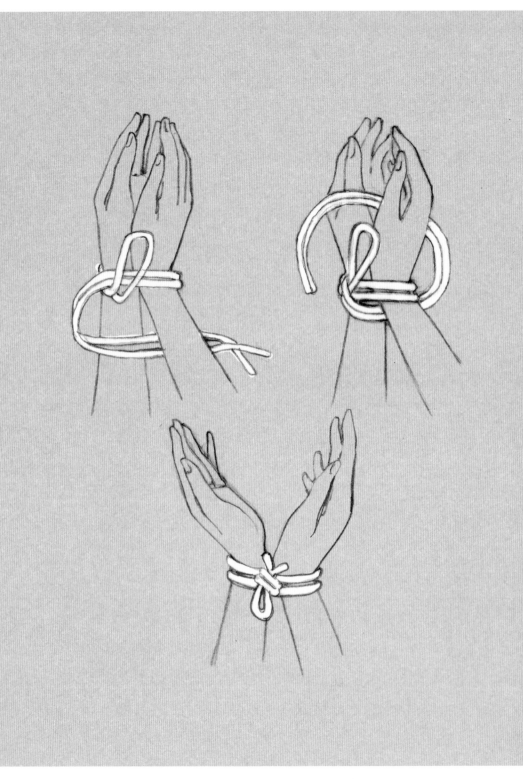

PLATE XII THE BASIC SHIBARI RESTRAINT

gradual mounting of sexual tension into the highest peaks of mutual pleasure; and ends with a slow "coming down" from the sexual high, which transforms into deeply intimate shared bonds and satisfaction.

SHARING YOUR GENEROSITY: INITIATING

The benefits of the Paradise Found Sexual Ceremony cannot be overstated. Nourishing the vitality of the libido regularly and in a ritualized context unites lovers and revives the luster and spontaneity of long-term monogamous relationships—evoking the beginning of the relationship and those precious hours stolen away in the service of ecstasy. The Sexual Ceremony has the power to reignite the spontaneity of the sexual vibration that first bound you together, as well as enforce the bond of new love. Making sexual satisfaction a priority is essential to the harmony, happiness, and longevity of all couples.

The easiest way to initiate a novice is to invite him or her to read the introduction to *The Boudoir Bible*, but the best way, if the laws of attraction haven't already gotten you in a frenzy, is to talk with the novice about the philosophy of the Paradise Found Sexual Ceremony. Few will argue with the generous nature of your ecstatic intentions—to accompany them on the discovery of the extent of his or her pleasure potential. But never try to force your ideas on anyone.

If a novice accepts your invitation, expound on the merits of your favorite tools and techniques. Be the example: voice your own needs and desires as well as your limits, and encourage your partner to do likewise. Listen and help him or her to overcome any embarrassment that communication about sexual matters can evoke, especially if physical or emotional limits are a concern. It will set a positive tone to the ritual, inspire trust, and put new partners at ease.

If the novice is a man, and you bring up the subject of ejaculation control, be prepared to explain why you shouldn't be misunderstood for an inconsiderate lover. The novice woman is less likely to object to the idea of being venerated at length. But in light of the fact that many women have "masculinized" their pleasure in order to adapt to the limitations of male sexual urgency, and others have yet even to experience orgasm, the need to explain the benefits of extended playtime remain, equally pertinent.

Whether one is a novice or experienced, personal limits change from day to day, from ritual to ritual, and from partner to partner; no single sexual encounter will ever be just like another. This is one of the many reasons for developing and refining sexual communication skills, and it is essential to a positive outcome, even when partners think they know each other well. The best time to share limits—physical, emotional, or even spiritual—is *before* the Sexual Ceremony begins. These "guidelines" for your partner may indicate that you don't wish to venture into anal territory, for example, or that you feel too vulnerable to be bound. Open, honest communication helps to ensure a heavenly ascent!

ANTICIPATION: THE CEREMONY OPENS

At the dawn of the Christian era, after the gods and goddesses of fertility, wine, and love were dethroned from the heavens, the concept of planning for sexual pleasure was likewise desanctified. The Paradise Found Sexual Ceremony brings the sacred back into sex, allowing us to create our own personal paradise where the stresses of everyday life, as well as the doldrums of everyday sex (or lack thereof!) can be transcended with profound sexual pleasure.

Most people consider great sex to be the ripe fruit of spontaneity and the idea of "planning" for pleasure synonymous with the extinction of the mysteries of sex. But in the context of the Sexual Ceremony, good planning is actually the fuel of spontaneity and inspiration.

Planning the ceremony a day or two days or even two weeks in advance is a potent form of psychological foreplay. It leads to sexual anticipation even before you and your partner have closed the doors on reality and commenced your ascent into the sexual dimension together. Planning ahead also permits you to thoughtfully clear away the reminders of everyday life, set the stage for the fulfillment of your desires, and prime your minds and bodies for the reception of pleasure. And then, once the curtains are drawn and the candles are lit, it is time to enjoy . . .

ABANDON YOURSELF: THE CEREMONY UNFOLDS

Lovers meet in the sacred space they have prepared with only one intention: to seek and provide sensual pleasure together. They abandon themselves to it, allowing the ceremony to progress in a crescendo of gradually more intense sensations focused on pleasure alone until a hypnotic "buzz"—an erotic trance—lifts them to ecstatic heights.

As in any ceremony, the Sexual Ceremony unfolds in phases, or sessions. These phases may be determined by a theme or a specific tool or technique, but they are always commanded by desire and unravel spontaneously through the ecstatic interaction of aroused partners. The ability of lovers to gradually heighten sexual tension through genital and extra-genital stimulation shapes the delectable rhythm of each phase. Worship the most plentiful source of the sexual vibration—the genitals—in alternation or in coordination with other erogenous zones of the body throughout the duration of the session. One of you may beg for more, but the limits established at the beginning of the ceremony must be respected. Women, explore your multiorgasmic capacity; men, ride the highest orgasmic wave over and over, until the pleasures become unbearable and crash over you, signaling the ending of the ceremony.

SATIATED LOVERS: THE CEREMONY CLOSES

The longer and more intense the journey, the higher lovers are likely to fly and the more time they will need to come down from the inebriating effects of endorphin elation. This culmination may be only one of many phases in the overall ceremony, or it may be the final "coming down" of two deeply satiated lovers. Taking the time to revel in the afterglow infuses the body, mind, and spirit with physical and emotional benefits.

Your descent from the heavenly heights will be as pleasurable as the ascent when you come down gently together—lying together, bathing each other, or preparing a ritual meal in preparation for your return to reality. Appreciate the moment—now that you have the keys to your personal Paradise, you may open that door together again whenever you wish.

CHAPTER 7

———o———

THE PLEASURE PRIORITY:
TIMING THE RITUAL

Out upon it, I have lov'd
Three whole days together;
And am like to love three more,
If it prove fair weather.

— "Constancy," John Suckling

BUSY PEOPLE ARE PRONE to convincing themselves that they "don't have time for sex." The time has come to set sexual satisfaction at the top of your to-do list; there is simply no more gratifying and effective way to counteract stress and lighten the pressure of heavy workloads while bettering the quality of your intimate relations! Whether you are living in the fast lane or managing a family with children, the real issue of time is not how little you have whittled down for personal pleasures but how you make the time for things that really matter.

REVEL IN THE RITUAL TEMPO

Time invested in the Sexual Ceremony is invaluable. When we are sexually appeased, we are in greater harmony with ourselves and, therefore, with our partners (and, for that matter, everyone around us). Our energy levels are higher, and we emanate a seductive, radiant glow as we move more positively through the world.

Asian philosophies of erotic loving can also be a source of inspiration. The Taoists suggest practicing the sexual union as often and for as long as possible, and Tantric texts encourage seven days and seven nights of erotic loving. While dedicating one whole day, much less a week, to the sexual ritual is rarely feasible in the real lives of most Westerners, deeply intimate and emotionally involved lovers who became skilled in the arts of the Sexual Ceremony find that doing just that becomes not only a possibility but also a pleasurable necessity—a Paradisiacal calling!

The Sexual Ceremony may last for as long as you wish, but prepare to dedicate a minimum of three hours for its elaboration. Though three hours may seem like too much time to invest in mere sexual revelry, in reality you will discover that it is just time enough to initiate and begin the unveiling of your body's pleasure potential. This being said, however, the Sexual Ceremony should never be treated as a test of endurance or a performance—it is a sacred voyage into the pleasure realm, a luxurious escape from reality.

To put the concept of a ritual tempo into perspective, as well as intent, consider the gradual unfolding of *Chaji*—the formal Japanese tea ceremony. Just like any other exquisitely perfect ritual, Chaji is organized thoughtfully in advance of the actual ceremony. Once the door of the teahouse has been shut with a bang to signal that all guests are present, the first phase of the ceremony commences. Before participants find their places, they admire the artwork that represents the chosen theme and helps set the tone of the ritual. A formal meal is served with three different kinds of tea. During the ceremony, the guests discuss and elaborate on the chosen theme, refraining from conversing about everyday life. Every element that is used to create this refined ritual, which can last for four hours or more, is carefully selected with the intent to guide guests into a timeless ritual dimension.

No matter how long a Sexual Ceremony lasts or how many phases comprise its ecstatic evolution, having an approximate idea of its duration before it commences will determine the manner in which the ritual space should be prepared, the range of tools and techniques that might be explored, and the intensity of the sensations that may be provided. The broader our sexual repertoires become, the more organic the extension of our ritual playtimes will be. Once we have learned how to abandon ourselves completely to the ritual dimension, the hours of pleasure will slip away ecstatically. Put aside sexual "goals" and revel in a timeless flow of adult playtime—the resulting sense of sexual satisfaction and deep fulfillment will radiate from within for days.

Whether lovers plan to transcend reality for a few hours or for a few days, forethought primes both partners—it is the prelude to greater pleasures than ever before experienced. The moment that the time, date, and place for the ceremony are confirmed, positive effects will begin to manifest. Clear your calendar, call the baby-sitter, and prepare to disappear into the temple (see plate XVII, page 275).

ESCALATING THE ECSTASY

The first phase of the ceremony actually commences when the time and date are confirmed. Preliminaries build anticipation even before the moment you actually unite with your lover. That tension alone may be enough to instigate your erotic worship when you finally come face-to-face in the temple of your choosing, but if you feel self-conscious or nervous at first, share a glass of champagne, a spicy drink, or a plate of fruit to initiate the ritual and help you shift into the ceremonial dimension. Make contact with your partner; if you or your lover are still tense or preoccupied with the worries of the world, relax with a massage while you talk about your erotic wishes: Will it be to explore a new tool or technique? To make love the good old-fashioned way? Or to engage in a light bondage session or tickle ritual?

Explore each other as if it is the first time you have ever had the privilege to do so, and, above all, let your bodies guide you throughout the hours that constitute every tantalizing phase of the Sexual Ceremony. Once the ceremony has progressed, those lovers who enjoy testing and "pushing" their limits may choose to explore the potentially more intense sensations provided by techniques like bondage, erotic flagellation, temperature play (discussed throughout the chapters in "Transcendental Techniques"), and anal penetration (described in the chapter "The Anthems of Anal Sex: From Hygiene to Heavenly Pleasures"). There are no rules as to how the phases will evolve nor how long they last, but the final outcome of each session (and thus the Sexual Ceremony as a whole) will be blissfully bolstered if the sensations introduced escalate gradually to more intense variations. Unless your lover needs intense sensations in order to perceive pleasure, techniques that push limits should be reserved for the (very) well aroused and practiced once the ceremony is well under way.

If you are engaging in a longer ceremony and choose to explore full-body techniques with their respective tools, experiment with the sensational effects that are generated when lovers keep to one role, that of provider (the "top") or receiver (the "bottom") of sensations, for the duration of one of the phases that comprise the Sexual Ceremony. In a later session, partners may decide to alternate roles, once the bottom has reveled in and descended from the inebriating effects of his or her top's generosity. Do note that whether or not you decide to stick to roles for the duration of a session, providing too many sensations in the same session is likely to create more sensory confusion than pleasure, while exploring a given few sensations to their fullest extent will ensure that the ritual keeps its momentum. It is the quality of the sensations that counts, not the quantity.

The shorter the Paradise Found Sexual Ceremony, the more important it is to keep things simple and limit the intensity of the sensations to be explored. If you or your partner is a novice, refrain from the practice of more extreme techniques until you have developed a comfortable degree of trust in each other. And remember that sex is not a test of endurance, nor is it a performance!

Also important to remember is that the increased activity of the endocrine system caused by the crescendo of pleasure creates a surge of hormones and endorphins that not only heightens our perceptions and therefore our *joie du sexe*, but also alters our state of consciousness and therefore our decision-making capacities. So no matter how "naturally high" you become, how long you play, and how intense the ritual becomes, *respect the limits that you established at the start*. I guarantee this will keep erotic tension high, preserve mystery between new partners, and avoid your having any regrets once the ceremony is over. Respect for boundaries also increases the likelihood that partners will continue to explore and "push" their limits once again at a later date.

HARDER . . . SOFTER . . . DEEPER . . . FASTER: GUIDE YOUR LOVER

Being "in the moment" and aware of your lover's reactions is as much a part of being a good lover as being able to abandon yourself wholly to pleasure. Lovers who are mentally and physically present reap extravagant pleasures on their journeys to and from Paradise. Being aware of each other's responses and reactions is the best guide to Paradise Found!

If your lover is making you swoon, let him or her know. If there is a little something he or she can do to enhance your pleasure, don't be afraid to ask for it. Guide your lover, verbally and physically, if you need them to go harder . . . softer . . . deeper . . . faster.

Most of us were trained in our youth to suppress, control, and hide our emotions, especially when our feelings had anything to do to with sex. Therefore it is not surprising that many adults take this failure to communicate to bed. But while reading our partner's body language is important, nothing can replace clear and honest verbal communication throughout the progression of the Sexual Ceremony. Depending on the personality of your partner, you can be straight-forward or persuasively subtle; communication is an art, and sexual communication is a further refinement of this art.

When lovers are exploring more intense sensations, open com-munication prevents accidents, avoids emotional outbursts, and keeps both psychological and physical boundaries clear. It also allows partners to map out the sensual geography of each other's bodies. Staying informed on the changes in the landscape is crucial to the journey to enhanced pleasure.

When enticing your lover, and inevitably yourself, into the arms of ecstasy, remain aware of his or her responses to your ecstatic attentions. Make harmonious transitions from one body zone to another, as jumping haphazardly from one kind of stimulation or body zone to another at random will make it very difficult for him or her to focus on and enjoy the sensations that you are providing. According to the Taoist of loving, lack of control, lack of attention, and lack of harmony are all synonymous with lack of sexual skill. Giving—and receiving—pleasure requires mental focus.

When providing subtle or feathery sensations, especially if you are concentrating on one specific area of the body, avoid letting your lover slip into a state of sensory boredom by varying the degree of contact. In the case that your lover is already warmed up, and you have progressed to the administration of more direct or intense degrees of stimulation, you should be all the more aware of their response to your generous attention.

Alternate the rhythm and the degree of contact that you provide in accordance with response to make certain that the sensations are leading to ever more intense degrees of pleasure. If at any time your partner resists or rejects or even recoils from the sensations that you are providing, interpret it as a clear signal to lessen the impact of your strokes, slow down, or divert your attention to a less sensitized area of the body. If your partner melts under your touch and goes into an erotic trance, continue doing exactly what you are doing; let them soar on the transformative effects that deep pleasure bestows upon body, mind, and spirit.

When performed in the ritual context, the administration as well as the reception of sexual sensations induces a trancelike meditative state. But this transcendental quality is less likely to manifest if partners try to explore too many different kinds of sensations at the same time. By exercising restraint and limiting the number of tools, techniques, and sensations to be explored, lovers will avoid sensory confusion and the risk of breaking the erotic trance. Remember that building sexual tension to transcendental heights takes time, and the longer the sexual ceremony lasts, the more intense the sensations become, and the greater the final impact of your ritual endeavor.

During lengthy ceremonies, your bodies will naturally signal for intermissions. The time that you dedicate to recuperation might include acts of necessity, such as eating, bathing, getting a breath of fresh air, and even deep sleep—all crucial to the positive evolution of lengthy ceremonies. Tension and fatigue render us physically and psychologically less receptive to stimulation—when we are fresh, our sensory faculties are more tuned in and thus well disposed. Recuperation rituals should be considered in a ritualized context in order to perpetuate, not interrupt, the flux of the sexual vibration. Partners should refrain from the temptation to converse about the problems and worries of everyday existence. Doing so will disrupt the rapture of the ceremonial dimension.

Lastly, the higher lovers fly on the inebriating effects of Eros, the longer it will take them to come down from the body's natural love drugs. Allow sufficient time to descend from your endorphin high before returning to reality. This is essential to the positive outcome of the Sexual Ceremony.

PREPARING FOR PARADISE

One essential element in the elaboration of the Sexual Ceremony is the preparation of the body. A hygiene ritual can be performed to honor all of the senses and transform the body into the stage for sexual pleasure. Envision that you are preparing a canvas upon which to express the arts of ecstasy.

A hot bath, or a shower, which tends to be more energizing, helps to reduce inhibitions and heighten sexual self-confidence. The skin is the body's largest organ, and when dead cells are allowed to build up on its surface, they create a barrier that inhibits the body's capacity to purify itself efficiently through the skin's pores. Using an exfoliating mitt or sponge or a granulated scrub to clear the pores and prompt circulation to the skin's surface and so enhance the perception of touch.

Like no other method, the steam sauna will eliminate toxins from the body and establish an overall sense of cleanliness, physically and mentally. Dedicating an hour per week to yourself in the sauna will keep body, soul, and mind primed for the reception of sensations. Brave the cold showers or icy pools of water that are available in most spas, as they serve to enhance the circulation of blood throughout your body. When performed within twenty-four hours of the ceremony's commencement, the sauna will notably increase your receptivity to intimate contact.

Remember that whether or not you include anal pleasures in your play, anal cleanliness is a critical aspect of genital hygiene.

Anal health and pleasure merits a chapter of its own: "The Anthems of Anal Sex: From Hygiene to Heavenly Pleasures." Note that while the genital area perspires more than any other zone of the body, and proper hygiene is important, overzealous, aggressive, or too frequent cleaning with scented detergents is likely to cause irritation to this delicate area of the entire body.

When a longer ceremony is planned, bathing and showering can be integrated into its progression. The recuperative pleasures of washing may be shared, and it is a great way for new partners to discover each other intimately. Let every trace of reality be washed away as your partner's soapy hands glide over your body—then return the favor.

Whether the bathing is performed as an event, an initiation into the ceremony, as an intermission, or as a way to terminate a long day of sexual worship, try finishing up the ritual with a cold genital rinse. If that sounds too shocking, recall that cold water invites blood to circulate and so keeps the genitals toned and ready for action. Once you have patted your clean skin dry, stroke each other from head to toe with a hydrating lotion or body oil.

As perfume and other scented body products may camouflage your natural pheromones, I advise that neither those nor underarm deodorant be used during the ceremony. The underarms are delectable area of the body to explore with your mouth, and there are few things as distasteful and distracting than the taste and feel of deodorant on your tongue! Your "scent aura," secreted by various glands (a number of which reside in the genital area), is a natural aphrodisiac that is to be respected as a precious elixir for the magical phenomenon of attraction.

The way that we take care of our hands and feet is a reflection of our overall hygiene; personal hygiene rituals should regularly include attention to these extremities. Reflexologists, masseurs, and acupuncturists consider both hands and feet to be gateways to the entire body, so keep this in mind when you kiss and stroke your lover's extremities with erotic intent. They are charged with millions of nerve endings.

HAIR OR BARE?

Another preliminary that may be performed before you arrive in the temple is the removal of body hair. Most women depilate their legs and their underarms, as well as remove traces of facial hair, for aesthetic purposes. In addition to keeping beards in check, many men today remove hair from their backs and chest, and some have adopted what was once known as a predominantly female practice, that of pubic preening.

While not everyone practices hair removal, some people go as far as to remove all of the hair from their bodies. Pubic depilation has been used by many cultures, past and present, for aesthetic as well as for sanitary reasons. Pubic hair removal was once believed to prevent the transmission of parasites, as well as sexually transmitted disease. Though we know today that this is not true, pubic hair does create a tactile barrier and acts as a trap for love juices. Its removal, therefore, can evoke a sense of cleanliness and provide for increased sensitivity and more direct contact.

The preference for a shaved pubic mound is also known as "acomoclitism." While some men and women continue to prefer the "bush" effect that was popular in the 1970s, increasingly more women and some men find partial, if not total removal, of hair from the pubic mound and the surrounding areas sexually appealing.

Today there are more ways to remove hair from the body than the Greco-Romans ever dreamed of. Alongside the classic razor blade, there are a variety of foams, gels, creams, and waxes, as well as lasers and electrolysis to remove hair permanently. In North Africa, traditional steam baths often include an area dedicated specifically to hair removal. It is more often than not performed with a ball of honey and beeswax. The most primitive, painful, yet painstaking form of hair removal is tweezing. Most people would consider pubic hair removal with tweezers a form of torture, but some people enjoy the sedative effects that it provides once the initial adrenaline rush subsides. And, strangely enough, until the second half of the twentieth century, the plucking of "pubes" with tweezers was used as a treatment for hysteria!

Ladies who prefer the Brazilian hot-wax method of hair removal report heightened levels of desire afterward. Most women find the process excruciating, but they deal with it because the pain is momentary; others claim to reach orgasm during the process. Everyone's threshold for pain is different, and, like it or not, waxing leaves you feeling slick, silky, and ready for intimate attention.

Any method that pulls the hair away at its root, like waxing or tweezing, brings blood rushing to the surface of the skin, and this renders the area very receptive to touch. It might not be appropriate, however, to those with very delicate skin. Electrolysis and lasers are techniques that also do not suit those who suffer from hypersensitivity.

When pubic hair removal is performed in the context of the sexual ceremony, razors are the best solution. They can make a strong psychological impact, especially if the razor in question is an open, or straight-blade, razor also known as a cutthroat razor. Unless you are skilled and at ease with this tool in hand, however, do not use it on someone else, as it is a potentially dangerous instrument.

If you and your partner practice pubic preening as part of the shared pleasures of the sexual ceremony, the person to be shaved should lie on his or her back, with knees bent and legs open as wide as possible. The position will fully expose the vulva or the testicles and it serves to pull the skin of the genitals and the surrounding area tight, allowing for a particularly close and safer shave. The position is obviously a vulnerable one, and it could be a source of humiliation; some lovers may actually enjoy this aspect of the ceremonial shave, though others will not appreciate the emotions it evokes.

Preparing the body and mind for pleasure is sexually empowering, and ritual preening is a titillating part of the preliminaries or a rejuvenating intermission in the Sexual Ceremony. It dissolves inhibitions, fosters receptivity, and cultivates the heightened pleasures that lie ahead.

CHAPTER 8

———o———

EROS AND ORDER:
ERECTING THE TEMPLE

Treat things poetically.

— Ralph Waldo Emerson

ANOTHER ESSENTIAL element in the elaboration of the Sexual Ceremony is the construction of your temple of erotic loving. This involves both a physical location and a psychological and spiritual dimension. By exercising control over a specific place and its ambience, you will be creating your private refuge from the real world, a sacred oasis for love. No matter how you define it—as the temple, the boudoir, the playroom, the dungeon, or the sanctuary—within this space your most intimate rituals will come to fruition.

In the eighteenth century, Catherine the Great, the Empress of Russia, dedicated several secret rooms to her sexual endeavors within her palace in Pushkin, outside of St. Petersburg. She famously had great interest in and know-how concerning the powers of sex as well as politics. The recent surfacing of a small part of the Empress's erotic equipage now confirms its often-denied existence. In the 2003 documentary film *The Lost Secret of Catherine the*

Great, director Peter Woditsch hypothesizes that what remains of the precious artifacts of her ecstasy are hidden in the Vatican vaults, the world's most extensive erotic museum, inaccessible to the eyes of the public.

Most of us do not have a room to spare solely for amorous celebrations. However, with a bit of creative fantasy, any room can be transformed into a temple of erotic loving. To erect the temple is a potent form of psychological foreplay that permits a gradual detachment from everyday reality, both mentally and physically, which is essential to sexual surrender and will help set fantasy free. The more sophisticated the ritual is, the more prepared partners will want to be in order to confirm a sense of freedom, safety, and relaxation that will enhance your mutual sexual satisfaction.

First and foremost is privacy. Even a slight interruption may disturb the rhythms of a sacred ritual. Second, before the temple doors are closed and locked to the outside world, every element necessary to the ritual's harmonious progression should be acquired and set in place (see plate XVIII, page 276).

A specific area should be dedicated to the setup of your pleasure kit: tools, lubricants, condoms, and whatever else you and your partner enjoy. (If you use battery-operated tools, make sure the batteries are charged.) Attention to detail before the Sexual Ceremony commences ensures that the ritual will not lose its pace—and this attention will build anticipation and act as a potent form of foreplay if you focus your thoughts on the pleasures that lie ahead. Disorganization is not erotic; aside from cooling down a heated moment, it may evoke a sense of insecurity in the partner on the receiving end, especially when full-body sensations are being explored. Nothing breaks an erotic trance like a lover fumbling in a closet to find a missing toy.

Whenever the central element of the temple happens to be a bed, its linens, clean and crisp, should be folded down like a ceremonial invitation. But make it a point from time to time to move the focus away from a bed's cozy confines. From a sexual point of view, beds limit our range of positions by confining us to the horizontal; they can make for lazier, more lethargic lovers. Experimenting beyond the borders of the bed is likely to reveal some very pleasant surprises. This being said, there is still no better place for a rejuvenating catnap than between the sheets in the arms of your partner.

Established couples may decide to either take turns or share in the organization of the ritual space; partners who do not know each other well may not be able to erect the temple together, but they might at least agree in advance upon the tools and techniques to be explored.

THE HOME AS EROTIC TEMPLE

For the established couple, the home is the obvious environment in which to erect the erotic temple. While it has the advantage of providing a permanent stage for more elaborate rituals, allowing for greater control, it also presents a greater challenge—that of keeping everyday reality at bay. Partners will need to make certain that the stress, worries, and obligations of everyday life are not allowed to creep into the ritual dimension, especially once the ceremony has commenced.

Switch off all telephones; make excuses in advance to anyone, such as a close relative, who might be concerned when you don't answer a call. (They obviously do not need to know exactly why you will not be responding!) You do not need anyone stopping by unannounced "just to make sure you are okay." Take off your watches—it's time to ignore the demands that the ticktock of the stately clock impose upon our lives. Allowing your body, not the clock, to be your guide through every phase of the ritual will reinforce the ceremonial dimension; you are breaking the normal rhythm of everyday existence.

However, if a specific time frame must be respected, an alarm can be set to about thirty minutes before the ceremony's end, allowing partners a fair amount of time to revel in the afterglow of ecstasy. Return to reality together, and do not end on a rushed note.

Close any doors leading to rooms that are not serving the ritual. Objects that may interfere with or interrupt concentration on the erotic joys at hand (such as piles of bills or laundry) should be put out of sight. Evoke the innate beauty of nature in the temple with a gorgeous bouquet of flowers. Let the Sexual Ceremony bestow order upon your domain. The more control exercised in advance over your environment's elements, the more likely it is that you and your lover will be able to truly let go and enjoy. A clean and orderly environment is more conducive to creativity and shows both self-respect and consideration for your partner.

PACK YOUR "PLAY CASE"

Hotel rooms can provide an interesting erotic alternative to the home environment, having the advantage of being a degree removed from everyday reality. Their spaces are like a proverbial clean slate, therefore receptive to any mood or theme that you and our lover decide to set. When you book the room, request a bathroom with a tub. You will, of course, need to pack your "play case" in advance: if it makes you happy, throw in a box of chocolates and a bottle of champagne. Include a travel candle or two, as the lighting in hotel rooms is rarely erotic. If you do not have travel candles, cut swatches of colored fabric and fold them into your kit. Wrapping the lampshades in the room with the cloth will cast a warmer, sexier glow.

Once you have hung the "Do Not Disturb" sign outside the securely locked door, check whether there is a gap between the bottom of the door and the floor. If there is, roll up a towel and place it snugly over the crack. If you can still hear people chatting in the corridor, then you can be certain that they will also be able to hear you. Be respectful of your neighbors. If you brought along instruments that could make compromising noises, like crops or floggers, you will need to either restrain your strikes or refrain from their use completely. Otherwise, the hotel manager may be knocking at your door!

Erecting the temple beyond the comfort and privacy of the home can present interesting limits and may result in the discovery of new sensations that would otherwise have remained unexplored. Remember, there is a great deal to be learned from limits!

FROLICKING IN THE GREAT OUTDOORS

If you are a nature buff, you may find playing outdoors appealing, when weather permits. Dealing with or surpassing the limits of the great outdoors can be a fun challenge. The sight and scents of wildflowers in bloom, the musky perfume of mossy cushions, and the magic of sunlight penetrating the leaves to dapple the ground can transform anyone into a naughty nymph or satyr.

If you plan to turn a *déjeuner sur l'herbe* into a mythic frolic, make sure that you are on secluded property. Personal security is crucial to the outcome of the sexual ritual, no matter where it is elaborated. If you decide to celebrate your ceremony outdoors, you should do so on your own land, or on land belonging to a friend or organization that shares your good intentions. Public parks and gardens, no matter how big or wooded they may be, should never be the site you choose. No public environment is private enough.

Venerating each other outdoors requires that we be aware of fauna and even flora that might be lurking. The lack of control that we have over Mother Nature can render outdoor ceremonies more complicated—no one welcomes scorpions, snakes, ticks, or bears in the ritual space. Nor does everyone enjoy the nonconsensual sting of nettles! Many complications can be avoided by simply being attentive to your surroundings.

If you are unable to completely guarantee privacy, comfort, and safety, but you have the privilege to be close to nature's embrace, in the course of a lengthy Sexual Ceremony you might wish to take your "intermissions" outdoors. Pack a picnic, or take a walk in the woods. It will give you the chance to become fully aware of the effects of your heightened levels of pleasure. Breathe deeply, and allow the sexual vibration to flow into and regenerate your entire being before you return to your indoor temple.

Whether the final aesthetic of the temple has elements of nature, Zen austerity, gothic moodiness, baroque grandeur, or is simply hard-edged modern, the space should reflect the sexual palates of both partners. As in the hermetic temples of the teachers of ancient Tantric disciplines, the atmosphere of a space can be designed to transport you straight from reality into your sexual dimension. The longer and more sophisticated the ritual, the more attention to preparation is desirable. Though at first this preparation may seem time-consuming, once lovers have refined their ceremonial skills, all the many tasks associated with preparing for the Paradise Found Sexual Ceremony will become highly enjoyable and even natural.

Keep in mind that the more intense a sexual ritual is, the more likely the participants are to experience long-term elation, the effect of the endorphin high. After ceremonies that have lasted for more than a few hours, venturing into reality may be slightly disorienting. Take as much time as you need to "come down" (driving on a "sexual high" or mingling with ordinary folk in supermarkets while under the effects of the erotic trance will do nothing to sustain those ecstatic rhythms). In the aftermath of the euphoric state, be aware that you may feel slightly estranged from reality, but that will reveal just to what extent you have flown on the wings of Paradise.

CHAPTER 9

———o———

ASCENT TO PARADISE:
ORCHESTRATING THE SENSES

The way you make love is the way God will be with you.

— Rumi, *The Book of Love*

THE TEMPLE OF your ritual space has been erected, and you are ready to close the doors on reality. You've prepared not only your body, mind, and spirit, but the ritual space as well, to fully honor each and every sense and thereby each other.

Pull the curtains closed, and light a candle or incense to signal the beginning of the ceremony. Incense has been used in many cultures to purify temples, and whether you choose frankincense, myrrh, or floral notes, its sacred accent will lead you toward the ritual dimension. Use essential oils as well as scented candles for erotic effect. The flames of candles cast magical, dancing shadows, and there is simply no one who does not become even more beautiful in their warm glow.

We tend to believe that our sense of touch is the most essential of the five senses to our pleasure, as it builds sexual tension faster than sight, hearing, smell, or taste. Catering erotically to every sense nourishes desire—the foundation of every creative impulse—as well as our perception of pleasures. The senses actually work best in unison, and the more they are strummed together with erotic intent, the more receptive to sensations we become.

A PAGAN FEAST FOR THE EYES

Men have been considered to be more visual than women, but in reality, for both sexes, the sense of sight is important in enhancing pleasure. It sparks desire, creates an intimate bond, and nourishes the flame of sexual passion throughout the duration of the sexual encounter. Unless you and your partner are reenacting a sexy medical scene that calls for bright light, turn the lights down low—but don't turn them off! Skilled lovers stay constantly aware of their partner's response to their loving attention, and this is simply impossible in the dark. If you cannot see the target of your passionate intentions or visually appreciate the beauty of their ecstasy, the lights are too low.

You have the ability to stop time in the temple. Create an eternal evening with soft, indirect light, even if the Sexual Ceremony commences while the sun is still high in the sky. This changes your perception of the passing of time, reinforcing the "otherworldly," ritual dimension of the ceremony. Wrap lampshades with scarves or fabric swatches, and further enhance the lighting by placing lamps on the floor, as indirect light from below is more atmospheric than from above.

Further delight the sense of sight with mirrors, considered by many to be the cornerstones of the temple's architecture. As bodies collide in paradisiacal rapture, large strategically placed mirrors will reflect a global vision of your ecstatic endeavors. Handheld mirrors tease with intimate close-up views. Mirrors evoke the thrill of group sex without presenting any of the real risks and unavoidable complications inherent to orgies. For the voyeur, mirrors are an excellent alternative to the use of pornography; they have the advantage of transmitting real sex, in real time!

And yet another word on the pagan feast for the eyes (and ears): pornography. We cannot pass through the visual realm without acknowledging that many people enjoy watching porn and use it as a potent audiovisual aphrodisiac, as well as an effective way to jump-start sexual desire. Pornography can be an effective point of ceremonial departure for some; for others, it keeps the sexual vibration from subsiding during an intermission.

If you use pornography, give it a proper place in the ceremonial context—in other words, don't let it take a front-row seat in the ritual space, as this is where you and your lover should be. The television screen is a modern pleasure-inhibitor, as there is nothing more frustrating than a distracted lover. If one eye is on you and the other on the screen, rest assured, your partner is fully dedicated neither to your pleasure nor his or her own. If you like porn, consider it "wallpaper in motion" or an ambient backdrop, turn off its audio and put on some sexy, sultry music in its place.

Appease the sense of sight with each and every detail—cleanliness and order delight the eye as much as beautiful materials do. Tools should be clean and arranged in an aesthetic invitation to play.

ECSTATIC HARMONIES FOR THE EARS

Music has been used to set the mood of nearly every ceremony that humankind celebrates, and the Paradise Found Sexual Ceremony is no exception. Music can inspire intimacy as it reinforces our physical, mental, and spiritual states. Choose music that will enhance the ceremonial mood, whether you commence dancing, performing a solo striptease, or, with no further ado, writhing together in ecstatic harmony.

Classical music relaxes the spirit and exalts the emotions. Before the ritual begins, turn down the volume of the music so that it melts into the background. This will not only heighten your concentration but also give precedence to the most beautiful songs of all, those we naturally make when the chords of ecstasy are strummed.

To repress these "songs of passion" is to perpetuate the Victorian myth that proper ladies and gentlemen should not audibly manifest sexual gratification. Refrain from taking this myth to bed, and your satisfaction will soar. As beautiful as the songs may be, they are likely to be interpreted as disturbing noise to those not playing a part in your symphony! If the temple is less than soundproof, playing music will create a sound barrier. Set the volume carefully to allow you and your partner to hear each other as well as mask your sighs and cries from the ears of next-door neighbors. By ensuring your privacy, it will enhance your sense of freedom.

As well as being a powerful aphrodisiac, the songs of pleasure that lovers spontaneously "sing" constitute a subtle erotic vocabulary. Breathing patterns alert the attentive lover to varying degrees of arousal. Short and fast breaths, accompanied by deep sighs and inarticulate *ummmm*s and *ahhhh*s indicate mounting sexual tension and a general state of receptivity. As breathing patterns become increasingly rapid, anticipate an imminent, cresting, orgasmic wave.

In the case of intense sensations being administered, however, a similar breathing pattern accompanied by the body's tensing, can be a sign that the sensory limits of your partner are being pushed. If he or she recoils, respond by decreasing the intensity or changing focus. A partner who passively submits to sexual play that he or she is not enjoying is as responsible as one who does not properly interpret a negative reaction; emotional if not physical distress will be the result.

Don't forget the beauty of the spoken word as an aphrodisiac! When you know what your partner best enjoys, tell him or her that you would like to give this pleasure. If your lover's response is positive, use the power of anticipation. Make him or her ask you in turn for it—or even beg! Anticipation has the advantage of prepping the brain, and your lover's mind will become intensely focused on the promised pleasure. When you finally provide the desired sensation, your lover will appreciate its effects all the more!

In any sanctuary, especially one of erotic loving, harsh tones and gestures break the mood of ceremony. However, when lovers delve into explorations of reenactment versus reality, the language of aggression may set the mood for certain forms of hierarchical role-play. For example, in the context of a consensual sexual scenario that entails power play—doctor/patient, teacher/student, master/servant—ritualized verbal aggression may be the appreciated prelude to an erotic discipline. This is explored further in the chapter "The Joy of Play: The Roles of Provider and Receiver."

INTIMATE APHRODISIACS

The language of love and food share the same tongue. A candlelit dinner is often the prelude to sexual revelry. The level of sensory excitement kindled by a beautiful meal strokes the libido, particularly if those savoring the oysters or cracking the lobster's claws have more intimate plans for the evening. Taking your taste buds into account is an excellent preliminary ritual, an ideal intermission, or a ravishing way to terminate the Sexual Ceremony. Preserve and promote the culinary arts and the related rituals of the table. Like the art of loving, this should be considered a priority for us all.

If the ceremony is due to last, place bowls of delectable, nutritious delights at fingers' reach. A few tasty examples of nutritional energy sources that will help partners maintain their stamina are fresh fruit, dried fruit, nuts, candied ginger (which cleanses the palate, enhances circulation, and rejuvenates), and chocolate.

Chocolate has long been associated with rituals, sex, and sentiments, and it is a perfect accompaniment to the Paradise Found Sexual Ceremony. Science is still trying to unwrap the mysteries that surround the sexy, dark brown delight that makes us feel so good. Research reveals that cacao naturally contains alkaloids like tryptophan and phenylethylamine, which trigger neurotransmitters in the brain. Neurotransmitters carry electrical messages between nerve cells, altering the way we feel and perceive sensations. The presence of phenylethylamine has also been tracked in the bloodstream of individuals who are in the state of falling in love! Like tryptophan, it incites a vertiginous feeling of excitement, elation, and happiness. The brain uses tryptophan to incite the production of serotonin—one of the body's natural antidepressants and yet another biochemical explanation for the "chocolate high."

In the context of the Sexual Ceremony, use it to tantalize the taste buds, provide energy, and reinforce your sexual high. Enjoy dark chocolate, containing at least 55 percent cacao, with known health benefits, instead of milk chocolate and refined-sugar candy disguised as chocolate.

When the ceremony is organized to last more than three hours, there needs to be more on the menu than snacks. While dining out is a good way to take an intermission, it has the disadvantage of removing you from the temple. Over extended periods of playtime, you will probably be more inclined to stay within the ceremonial dimension. Nutritious and aesthetically pleasing meals can be prepared, at least partially, in advance. Cooking a ritual meal for your lover is another way to make love to him or her. Whether you dine out, order in, or prepare your ceremonial meals at home, the menu should always be made of light, fresh, high-energy foods that are nutritious and easy to digest.

Lovers will notice that their sense of taste will be accentuated over extended periods of sexual arousal. In order to further enhance the positive progression of your sensorial voyage, choose ingredients that have sex appeal. Some foods traditionally known to nourish the libido are truffles, oysters, fish roe, and chili peppers. The psychological impact that certain foods have is often higher than any actual sexual enhancement they might supply. This explains why phallic-shaped foods, like the banana or zucchini, or the yoni-shaped fruit of the strawberry, are considered to be aphrodisiacal. Still, the greatest aphrodisiac of all is providing pleasure and receiving it in return.

I recommend that certain foods be avoided altogether: pasta, bread, or fried foods, or any food lurking under heavy cream sauce or smothered in cheese. These foods demand too much energy to digest and will leave you feeling lethargic. Limit your consumption of carbohydrates, and indulge in light, fresh foods in small portions. It is always advisable to eat less, it will enhance the evolution of the ritual to feel energized and ready for action once you're up from the table.

Some ingredients are best avoided unless both partners consume them, for example, onions and garlic. While these less-than-delicate but delicious delights are considered to be aphrodisiacal, they are also renowned for causing very bad breath. If, however, garlic or onions are consumed in good company, their sexual unappeal will become barely perceptible, and you are less likely to offend each other.

When celebrating your ceremonial endeavors with a glass of champagne, forget the not-so-bubbly idea of utilizing the bottle to penetrate your lover for fun—either before or after you pop the cork. If it is sealed, agitating a bottle of champagne (in combination with the temperature change provoked by the warmth of the human body) may cause the contents to explode, which could be detrimental to your lover, to say the least! Also, if the bottle is already opened, inserting it inside the vagina or anus can create a vacuum effect that is equally dangerous.

Be very discerning about what you put or allow to be put inside your body, and keep in mind that the mucus membranes of the vagina and the anus quickly transmit into the bloodstream any substance that they come into contact with. In addition, inserting food into the vagina presents the risk of vaginal yeast infections. Yeast thrives on substances that contain sugar, and so the erotic classics of honey, chocolate, strawberries, and ice cream inserted into the vagina may induce such an infection. Serve dessert on a plate to avoid the risk.

It is also for this reason that alcohol should never, ever be poured into the anus or the vagina, as it will induce an instant state of inebriation (a possibly unbecoming side effect). Alcohol can also irritate the linings of both vagina and anus.

SEX, DRUGS, AND ALCOHOL—OR NOT

This leads us to a topic of great relevance—sex, drugs, and, alcohol. Both amphetamines and alcohol excite our senses and liberate us from our inhibitions, but both substances are also vascular constrictors that reduce rather than encourage the blood flow to the genitals. Contrary to popular belief, alcohol and other drugs inhibit rather than heighten our sensory perception and therefore negatively influence our capacity to experience truly deep levels of sexual satisfaction. They also mask the positive effects of endorphin elation; endorphins, unlike drugs and alcohol, increase our overall sensorial perception and therefore the effects of the orgasm.

Endorphins not only make us feel good, but they are good for us, too. Unlike other mind-altering substances, endorphins do not produce negative effects on the mind or body.

The best way to accentuate their effects is to drink plenty of water throughout the duration of the Sexual Ceremony. Add an elixir of ginseng to your carafe to create an alcohol-free energy booster. Because ginseng is a stimulant, it should not be consumed in the evening unless you and your partner plan to play all night.

Even though the Italians declare that a glass of red wine per day keeps the heart healthy (and the French are the first to concur), alcohol should be consumed with moderation during the Sexual Ceremony. While a single cocktail, a glass of wine, or a flute of champagne can have a positive effect on the psyche and help a tense lover to relax, large quantities of alcohol will radically limit your perception of pleasure and alter your sense of judgment. Its effects may make you forget your limits, emotionally as well as physically. No one wants to wake up from an evening of bacchanalian delight with sex-related regrets caused by a void in the memory! Alcohol can also hinder the male erection and cause vaginal dryness by depleting the Bartholin's glands of lubricating mucus. Alcohol has a dehydrating effect on the entire body. Antihistamines can also produce this effect, although the discomfort that dryness provokes during penetration can be counteracted through the use of lubricants.

Like alcohol, tobacco is also a noted vascular constrictor. It can have a negative effect on the male erection, on the impact of our orgasms, and upon our libido. Tobacco is also known to affect the vitality of sperm, decrease their production in the testicles, and finally, limit the volume of the fluids that are emitted during ejaculation. Tobacco also produces unpleasant odors that will linger in the ritual space. While smokers may not be susceptible to these odors, most nonsmokers are. Try to refrain from smoking in the temple. Incense and other home fragrances may camouflage bad odors, but they will not eliminate their cause.

There is no need to dwell further here on the negative effects that nicotine and other drugs and alcohol heap upon our entire organism—including our capacity to experience heightened degrees of sexual satisfaction. The well-executed Sexual Ceremony is a "drug" in itself, one that is healthy, legal, and free to all who embark on the journey to Paradise.

TITILLATING TOUCH

Making love is about all the senses, but touch remains one of the most powerful and versatile paths to pleasure. In establishing contact with your lover, you can provide titillation and excitement or convey security and trust. Touch has the power to initiate the Paradise Found Sexual Ceremony, to signal changes in phases, or to provide a blissful way to "come down" after extended pleasures.

A massage is a divine way to initiate intimate contact, especially if your partner is not quite ready and is perhaps tense or preoccupied. An erotic massage will permit you to back off yet continue to transport your lover into the sexual realm, such as during an intermission. It is also an excellent way to get a sensory overview of the sensual landscape. If you feel insecure about administering massages, read about the subject, or take a class to help you build confidence and develop some skills. Getting a massage is also great way to learn how to give a massage.

An effective massage can be performed without a lot of complicated techniques; let your creative energy flow, and follow your instincts. If you invite your lover to tell you what he or she desires, you will gradually find yourself able to give a very effective and personalized massage.

Try beginning with a head massage. The head is home to four of our five sensory organs and also houses the biggest sexual organ of all, the brain. A head massage has the power to lead even the most nervous of lovers toward a more receptive state.

Massage the top and the back of the head. Gently pull the hair to invite blood to rise toward the surface and freely circulate. Rub and then kiss the place between the eyebrows known as the third eye. This area, highly receptive to the transmission of energy, is the door to the inner spirit.

Carefully kiss the sensitive eyelids. Massage and kiss the ears, charged with nerve endings that will transmit ripples of erotic sensation throughout the entire body. Kiss and bite the neck of your lover with erotic intent, to send similar waves of erotic energy up his or her spine.

The heavy muscles of the buttocks, thighs, upper arms, and the back are responsive to deep and penetrating pressure. Though not as sensitive or sexually charged as other areas of the body, for this reason they are a good starting point for erotic contact. (Unless you are a truly skilled masseur, the spinal column should be avoided.)

As you massage, always work in the direction of the heart. Imagine that you are literally pushing the blood back toward its vital source, and the effects of the massage will be more rejuvenating. You don't want your lover to fall asleep! Whether your massage is a prelude to, or an intermission in the sexual ceremony, intermittently stimulate the genitals. Toward the end of the massage, experiment with ways to provide more and more contact between your body and that of your lover, taking the ritual to the next level.

Massage oil or talc will render the massage easier for the provider, but remember that neither is conducive to vaginal or anal health. Latex gloves can be worn to add a sensory twist to the manual administration of sensations, as long as you are not using oil, which causes them degrade. Talc on latex gloves, however, will exalt the effects of the massage. Or try wearing only one glove, the other hand bare, providing two different sensations simultaneously.

Leather gloves are sexy, and permit the provision of deep, penetrating sensations, but they also create a certain resistance. So if you plan to conserve your energy, they are not the best option. Leather gloves also have a disadvantage of reducing the direct exchange of energy from the receiver's body to the provider.

Men, use your genitals to offer a hot, deep, and even slightly funny massage by rolling your erect member back and forth over the back, the thighs, and other zones of your lover's body. (The pleasure is obviously shared!) Ladies, finish off your massage by guiding your nipples over your lover's skin. From this, too, the masseuse will enjoy a degree of auto-stimulation.

While the hands are the body's most effective tactile instruments, remember that the mouth—the lips, tongue, and teeth—also can provide deeply intimate pleasure. Along with the anus and vagina, the mouth represents the only other round muscle in the body, and it is similarly composed of highly sensitive erectile tissues. Nerve endings are clustered all through the mouth area, which is why it feels so good to kiss, nibble, caress, suck, lick, and taste each other. While a kiss on the lips is divine, when tongues come together, lovers are likely to be led toward even greater sensory pleasures. The lips can be used to kiss and caress any part of the body. The tongue happens to be one of the strongest muscles in the human body, and when used artfully, it elicits sensations that no other part of the human body can provide.

The Taoist disciplines of erotic loving suggest a series of exercises to reinforce the mighty muscle of the tongue, in order that it may be used to provide oral pleasures at length. The teeth, on the other hand, can be used to test the limits between pain and pleasure. While not everyone appreciates the pungent sensations that love bites provide, the desire to lick, taste, and literally consume the one we love is an integral part of passionate love and a sign of great trust and intimacy.

CHAPTER 10

———o———

THE JOY OF PLAY:
THE ROLES OF PROVIDER
AND RECEIVER

There are two ways to reach me: by way of kisses or by way of
the imagination. But there is a hierarchy: the kisses alone don't work.

— Anaïs Nin, *Henry and June: From a "Journal of Love,"*
the Unexpurgated Diary (1931–1932) of Anaïs Nin

THE PARADISE FOUND Sexual Ceremony provides adults with the rare opportunity to play—switching off the real world and turning each other all the way on! Incorporating erotic play can help to determine the focus of the ritual's elaboration as well as facilitate the introduction of the tools and techniques of full-body stimulation.

Role-play is a natural and spontaneous aspect of every child's recreation—the imagination has no limits. At some point in our childhoods we all embodied adult roles, either the dominant or the subordinate role or alternating between them. Perhaps we played a heroic soldier, beating down a feeble enemy, or in turn, we were the enemy being overpowered by the conqueror. We may have been a pirate or the helpless captive, cop and robber, master and pet, a teacher with her naughty pupil. Role-playing gives the child the opportunity to explore the many juxtapositions of strength with impotence, according to the inclinations of a budding personality. But by the time we reach adolescence and begin to mature sexually, most of us have learned to judge the world of fantasy as childish, our social conditioning smothering the spontaneity of our creative minds. Ironically, once many of us attain adulthood and assume its chosen or imposed roles, we often worry more about what we should or should not do, say, think, or feel, rather than simply being ourselves and exploring our roles, whatever they may be, creatively.

Erotic play awakens the child-spirit that dwells deep inside every adult. Whether or not lovers develop specific roles, every sexual encounter inherently involves a degree of domination and submission on behalf of both partners. Great sex plays with and stretches the lines between pleasure and pain, whether lovers play hard or soft, or go so far as to create a scenario and develop specific characters. Spontaneous or premeditated, erotic play can help lovers to tap into and satisfy their deepest needs (see plate XIX, page 277).

READY & WILLING: TOPS & BOTTOMS

Lovers who enjoy BDSM play sometimes use the explicit terms "master" and "servant" to describe the roles of the provider and receiver of sensations. In the context of the Paradise Found Sexual Ceremony, I prefer the words "top" and "bottom" (and the verbs "to top" and "to bottom") to describe the activities that correspond to giving and receiving sensations.

"To top" is to provide undivided sexual attention to a ready and willing bottom. "To bottom" means to accept and thereby submit to and enjoy the sexual stimulation provided by the top. These do not have to be strict categories but are instead roles to be assumed as you desire with your partner. Unlike BDSM activities, in which partners are often expected to assume and stay with only one role, that of dominant or submissive (an individual who alternates between these roles is sometimes derogatively known as a "switch"), within the Paradise Found Sexual Ceremony, partners are encouraged to alternate between the roles of top and bottom and even to switch between these roles during the same ritual. After all, if we don't submit to pleasure, we cannot tap into and reap its powers.

That being said, creating sexual ceremonies around specific roles is certainly not forbidden. When the duration of the ceremony is limited, lovers may wish to develop well-defined roles within specific scenarios. This is particularly relevant if techniques like bondage and flagellation are to be explored, because these require higher states of arousal in order for the sensations to be interpreted as pleasurable. Then, the next time you play, try inverting your roles. However, far better is to create time in your schedules for a longer ceremony that will allow you to top and bottom each other all the way to Paradise and back, over and over again!

No matter how many times you and your partner spontaneously switch roles during a given ceremony, avoid playing the same role at the same time—two bottoms will make for a sluggish ceremony, while two tops may risk creating more conflict than reciprocal ecstasy! Keep in mind that a satisfied bottom will be all the more willing to invert the roles and in turn take gracious care of a generous top-turned-bottom.

TAKE COMMAND

Skilled tops aim to administer sensations in harmony with their bottom's needs and desires. No matter how lovers attain sexual satisfaction, the limits of the partner who is bottoming should determine the parameters of the Sexual Ceremony's progression. But while the bottom's role is to submit to pleasure, this does not imply that he or she is passive. The generation and exchange of sexual energy is a joint effort, and the bottom is equally responsible for the outcome of the Sexual Ceremony. Like a skilled top, a skilled bottom leaves the world behind and drops into a truly relaxed and receptive mental and physical state of readiness. A bottom interacts with his or her top constantly, concentrating fully on the pleasures being provided.

A skilled top remains similarly aware of and responds accordingly to the bottom's reactions. A bottom's body language should be enough to indicate whether the top is doing something too fast, too hard, too tight, too light, not quite right, or perfectly well! If a bottom slips into a relaxed and receptive state, it is a good indication that he or she appreciates the top's attentions and is already on the way to Paradise.

A bottom's resistance to any form of contact, on the other hand, should be interpreted as a clear sign that he or she does not perceive the sensations that are being administered as pleasurable or acceptable. If a top fails to respond correctly to this kind of body language by backing off, altering focus, or changing the tool or technique being used, the bottom should tell the top calmly what is interfering with his or her sense of satisfaction, or even interrupt the ritual.

The potential pleasures of erotic play can be explored by integrating role reversal into the Sexual Ceremony. For example, women may assume the upper hand (which some still associate with the man's role). If you normally prefer to bottom, learning to top through role reversal is likely to reveal surprisingly empowering effects. Take command! Undress your lover, and do not consider getting undressed until he or she is totally naked. Then, when you do strip down, work the erotic powers of anticipation and mystery. Take your time.

In a similar vein, switching is an effective way for lovers, both male and female, to discover the merits of fully accepting and submitting to pleasure. Women especially have been culturally programmed to provide, not only as mothers but also as lovers. They may, therefore, have more difficulty accepting the gift of pleasure than men. But assuming the bottom's role reduces performance pressure, allowing lovers, male or female, to lie back and accept their innate right to be pleased and truly let go. Remember that your pleasure is your partner's pleasure!

ACT OUT

Lovers who feel uninhibited about the idea of erotic play may enjoy the reenactment of defined roles within the parameters of specific fantasies. Do not be surprised if your adult fantasies are similar to those associated with both BDSM and child's play. Roles that juxtapose power or the lack thereof are archetypical, remaining the same from generation to generation. Such erotic fantasies as being held captive or kidnapped, spanked like a schoolboy, pampered like a puppy, or taken care of by a nurse are in the collective unconscious and are familiar to all of us. However, you must first communicate your wishes and needs to your lover. Failure to do so before acting out your fantasy could get you kicked out of the boudoir!

You may enjoy fantasy-driven playtime that stages the physical and emotional effects of fear, anger, or elation in order to explore an ever-wider range of sensations and emotions during erotic playtime. When emotions are acted out within the boundaries of a specific fantasy with a trusted lover in a controlled and protective environment, they are likely to incite the "sexual high."

Ritualized vulnerability, humiliation, and even aggression, whether verbal or physical, can be integrated into the ceremonial context as long as both partners consent and the session evolves harmoniously within predetermined and very precisely defined parameters. You should never feel obliged to take part in any sexual activity with which you do not feel perfectly comfortable, and erotic playtime should never evolve in a less than loving and attentive fashion.

Acts of genuine aggression or violence during any form of sexual encounter, much less the Sexual Ceremony, should be considered abuse and not be tolerated. To intentionally threaten the physical or emotional well-being of anyone is neither acceptable nor compatible with the philosophy of the Paradise Found Sexual Ceremony.

The exploration of roles that correlate to the emotional and physical impact of *ritualized* fear, aggression, or danger, conjoined with sexual arousal, should always be elaborated in extremely controlled environments. Remember that reenactment is not reality, but if outsiders should hear, much less witness, a scene that pushes sexual boundaries, they could mistake the actions for real abuse. The erotic temple is organized *ad arte*, and every ecstatic improvisation should progress in total privacy.

Those who practice more intense forms of stimulation while reenacting specific roles might consider the improvisation of loose scripts, especially if it is the first time that they play together. Defining the limits of the ritual in advance will also help lovers safely guide each other from the real world into the sexual dimension with greater ease.

BDSM role-play often implies elaborately defined scripts, with lines, ritual expressions, and specialized terminology to make the re-creation of a specific scene more "realistic." This is also common practice among professional dominants. Because they practice often with people they do not know well or at all, they may also make use of written negotiations or contracts in order to learn as much about the person they are playing with as possible. This form of negotiation is an example of how good communication serves to guarantee erotic satisfaction. Whether they are written or verbally negotiated, creating boundaries will avoid placing either partner in unnecessarily awkward positions.

GET DRESSED TO UNDRESS

The use of specific props enhances the physical, psychological, and aesthetic impact of the ritual as a whole. Props also permit lovers to execute the ritual more coherently and with conviction. Costumes can also be used to render the realm of fantasy more realistic. They reinforce the effects of specific roles and make for even greater fun. After all, if you really want to be worshipped like a god or a goddess, you need to make an effort to get dressed (and undressed!) like one.

Let's take the corset, for example. If a woman were to dress in a corset, she'd find that it disciplines her curves, reduces her waistline, and lifts her breasts, thereby making a very composed and poised statement. First developed in the Middle Ages, the corset has undergone many transformations over time, but it has never fallen completely out of style. At the beginning of the nineteenth century, even men's fashions called for stays, which were used to emphasize the waistlines and punctuate the torsos of military officials and dandies. Today some men still use stays, more or less secretly. The corset enforces good posture, changes the way we move through space, and empowers the wearer by heightening body awareness.

Corsets may be used to enhance the elaboration of many role-playing scenarios, from military scenes with a disciplinary slant to Great Goddess worship. Those who choose to explore more extreme degrees of constriction and assume the classic hourglass shape (that a steel-boned corset can best provide) will need assistance—not only in getting properly laced into the corset but also in performing any task that requires bending forward, such as tying shoes. Extreme corseting is performed in two or three phases over a period of at least thirty minutes in order to permit the inner organs to rearrange themselves around the constriction.

High heels and lingerie are probably the most readily accepted of female erotic accessories, and most men are subject to their powers of seduction. Slipping into something silky, sheer, and provocative is as sexy as getting slipped out of it. Fine stockings define the legs and create a veiled promise of pleasure, whether your perfectly manicured feet are sliding into, or out of, a pair of dizzyingly tall high-heeled shoes. Like corsets, high heels change the way we move through space. The provocatively shod are sexually empowered . . . and empowering!

The erotic appeal of leather tantalizes through the senses of sight and touch, but its distinctive creak and musk are also a turn-on for those who appreciate these materials—as is the squeak, snap, and slap of latex for rubber aficionados.

The more specific the erotic play becomes, the more precise the costumes and accessories can be. Erotic fantasies involving the police, the military, doctors, nurses, firemen, and serving maids become much more exciting and realistic when their related uniforms are worn. They are an effective way to add a little spice and a lot of entertainment to any sexual encounter. The possibilities to enhance the quality of our sexual playtime become endless when we think outside of categories.

No matter what roles lovers assume, costumes, tools, and props reinforce the ritual dimension by making adult playtime more convincing, aesthetically appealing, and fun. When practiced with creative gusto between consenting, uninhibited, and creative adults, reenacting specific scenarios within predetermined parameters will evoke sensations and emotions that would otherwise probably go undiscovered. This experience is not an obligation, but its liberating effects can incite physical as well as emotional and spiritual transformations and thrust open doors to a more adventurous and fulfilling life, and not just within the boudoir alone.

PART III

———o———

TRANSCENDENTAL TECHNIQUES

In which the tools of desire
that bring lovers to the heights of Paradise
and beyond are revealed.

THE CHAPTERS THAT FOLLOW are an initiation into some of the most
creative and sexually empowering techniques of full-body stimulation.
They invite lovers to explore erotic frontiers beyond the genitals
and engage the entire body—and mind—as a sexual, sensual whole.
Many people refuse to explore these techniques because of fear of
physical risks, but more do so out of fear of being categorized S&M,
or judged as perverted or "abnormal."

Sexual categories create impediments. The chapters within "Transcendental Techniques" explore sexual potential; once lovers tap into the possibility of shedding the fear of judgment, they begin to see beyond these artificial boundaries and overcome physical, emotional, and even spiritual blocks to experiencing and sharing greater sexual pleasure.

Here it must be reiterated: there is no right or wrong or even "normal" way to make love—as long as the means that lovers take to experience satisfaction do not infringe upon the desires, rights, or the innocence of anyone involved. To refuse to experience novel sensations for fear of being judged is to refuse the possibility of discovering deeper dimensions of yourself and your lover or lovers, as well as the wider world of pleasure that the sexual union can and should represent.

But even if you choose not to explore these admittedly different yet physically and psychologically enlightening options, refrain from immediate judgment. Read on to broaden your perspective. This may permit you to reevaluate humanity's differences, which are at the heart of what makes every one of us so wonderfully unique.

CHAPTER 11

———o———

EXPANDING THE SEXUAL ARENA: IMPLEMENTS OF ECSTASY

I am made for love . . . from head to toe.

— Marlene Dietrich, *Der Blaue Engel*

I USE THE TERMS "instruments," "tools," "scepters," and "implements of desire" rather than "sex toys" to describe the objects that permit lovers to provide sensations in the sexual arena. Though the Internet has put an end to the days when lovers were obliged to shop underground or on the wrong side of town for whips, restraints, or other creative implements of desire, this accessibility is not yet synonymous with acceptability. Similarly, though many of these accessories, once condemned as S&M or "fetish," have come to be considered fashionable, glossy magazines and designer labels have done little to change the way most people judge erotic tools and those who use them.

Exploring sexual frontiers with the aid of erotic implements, particularly those that serve to stimulate the body and not the genitals, continues to be identified with the darker side of sex. This distorted image is perpetuated by the media and film industries, which associate behavior that goes beyond the stereotypical portrayal of PGO sexuality with perversion or criminality—and, basically, what viewers have been led to believe is what they expect to see. Most producers of so-called sex toys involuntarily reinforce these negative viewpoints and perpetuate the taboo of extra-genital stimulation by failing to accompany their products with instructions for their correct, safe, and pleasure-enhancing use. Like any tool, sexual instruments must be used with know-how in order to yield positive results. Sexually evolved Taoist and Tantric practitioners (as well as their modern devotees, who use sex to transcend reality and come closer to the divine) looked upon any instrument that permitted them to explore and push the limits of the sexual realm not as a toy but as an object of power.

To put erotic instruments into perspective, consider the most powerful and versatile sexual implements we have: our hands. Mother Nature equipped us with not one or two but a total of ten digits, thus ten times the potential to provide ecstasy. When used skillfully, the hands can undress, heal, caress, stroke, spank, hold, tickle, and massage the ones we love to love. When used carelessly, they can also inflict pain and injury. As is the case for any erotic implement, it is the manner and the context in which the hands are employed that make the difference between the providing joy or distress, ecstasy or agony.

Tools of desire are simply extensions of the hands (and in some cases, extensions of other parts of the body), and they should be used with the same guidelines—respectfully and in harmony with each individual's desires, level of skill, and intent to pleasure. Ticklers, crops, and restraints provide sensations similar to those that can be performed with the hands—tickling, slapping, and holding—while tools like whips and floggers help lovers provide sensations that would otherwise be complicated, if not physically impossible, to administer with the hands. Like every tool, from a hammer to a computer, these erotic instruments should be viewed as aids. They simply have the ability to provide sensations more effectively than our hands, and if partners so desire, more intensely and at greater length.

Tools expand our sensorial repertoires and allow us to stroke the pleasure centers of the brain in new and different ways. Techniques like erotic tickling, restriction, constriction, and flagellation can be used during the Paradise Found Sexual Ceremony to engage the whole body over extended periods of skillful and creative stimulation, triggering the steady release of pleasure-enhancing endorphins and hormones while coaxing sexual energy to radiate outward from the genitals. When extra-genital pleasures are combined or alternated with genital stimulation, the entire body, as well as the mind and spirit, becomes charged with sexual vibration.

In addition to granting access to higher dimensions in the sexual realm, erotic tools offer an aesthetic value in the context of a sexual ritual. Aesthetics are pertinent to the positive outcome of any cere-mony—from High Mass to an English or Japanese teatime to the Paradise Found Sexual Ceremony. The potency of any ceremonial object relies upon the manner in which the participants interact with the object and share in its empowering potential. The design of the tools and the quality of their materials reinforce the difference between ritual and reality.

TO EACH HIS OR HER OWN

A common misconception about sexual tools is that they are only used to inflict pain. But these same instruments can also give subtle, sensuous stimulation. Remember that what one lover may consider painful may very well be another lover's Paradise. Everyone has a different perception of pleasure. Similarly, everyone also has a dif-ferent threshold for pain; some people need intense sensations in order to perceive pleasure and experience sexual satisfaction. This transformation of pain into sexual arousal is known as "algolagnia."

Those who practice this approach to satisfaction are not seeking to be injured but, on the contrary, to be physically and emotionally

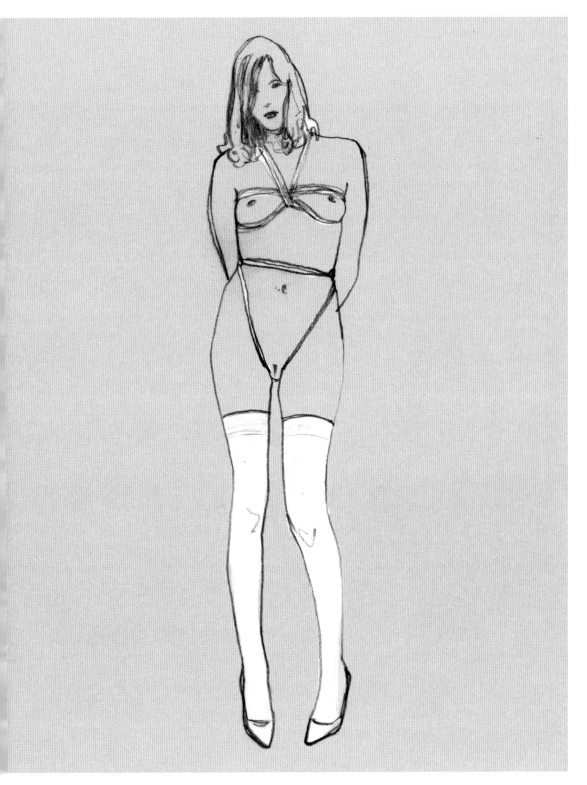

PLATE XIII THE CHEST HARNESS

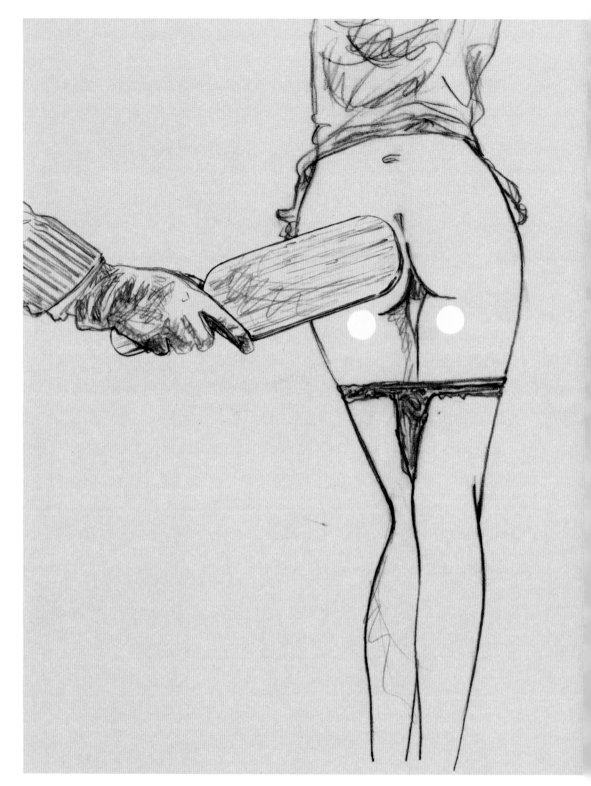

PLATE XIV SPANKING SESSION AND THE "SWEET SPOT"

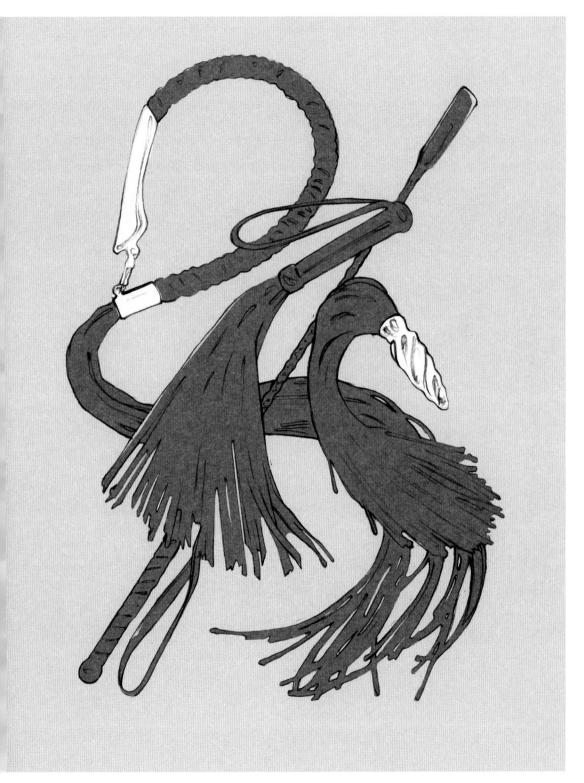

PLATE XV INSTRUMENTS FOR EROTIC FLAGELLATION

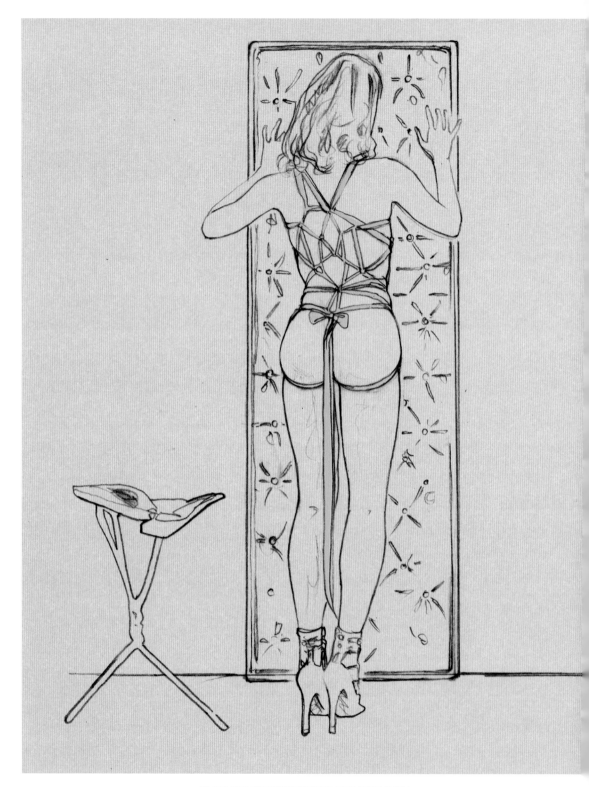

PLATE XVI THE UNKNOTTED TORTOISE SHELL

appeased, and they do not even necessarily consider themselves part of the BDSM realm. Similarly, those who do engage in BDSM relations are not necessarily only seeking to receive or provide pain. That every "servant" or "slave" is a masochist and every "master" or "dominatrix" is a sadist is another misconception. While some do adhere to the "no pain, no gain" philosophy of pleasure, others do *not* wish to provide or experience even the slightest effects of physical pain. Likewise, those who are sexually subservient and seek the psychological impact of being humiliated might fit the BDSM cliché to perfection; but in reality, not every "servant" is necessarily at ease with such games. To each his or her own!

Categories aside, those who revel in the powers of the tools and techniques of full-body stimulation appreciate their capacity to incite the sexual high. Techniques such as consensual erotic tickling, constriction, restriction, bondage, and flagellation create a surge of endorphins and hormones, including dopamine and oxytocin, just two of the bodies' many natural "love drugs." Several factors will contribute to this increased production, including the top's ability to provide sensations skillfully in a gradual crescendo, the bottom's degree of receptivity to these sensations, and the gradually growing intensity of these sensations over extended periods of arousal. The more partners are sexually attracted to each other, the more endorphins and hormones they naturally produce, and the greater the rewards of ecstasy are likely to be.

THE RAPTUROUS CRESCENDO

Endorphins, in combination with other inebriating chemicals that are produced and processed in the body during lovemaking, are the liaisons between pain and pleasure, between increasingly intense sensation and heightened degrees of sexual satisfaction. Some of these chemicals increase our resistance to pain while others heighten our sensory perception, including our perception of pleasure. This helps to explain why some individuals appreciate more extreme stimulations, and why, over longer periods of arousal, we are all able to take pleasure in increasingly intense sensations. That is also the reason why the intensity with which sensations are bestowed should always be orchestrated as a progressive crescendo, allowing for a gradual increase of pleasure-enhancing endorphins and hormones in the system.

If an intense sensation is given before sexual tension builds, and adequate endorphins have yet to seep into the system, it is likely to be perceived as pain, not pleasure, with an accompanying adrenaline rush. Produced in the adrenal glands, adrenaline is an essential ingredient in the hormonal recipe that incites the sexual "high." It also accentuates our perception of any sensation, pleasurable or not. When sensations such as fear, danger, and pain cause adrenaline production to spike, the self-preserving "fight or flight" response is triggered. Skilled tops coax the production of adrenaline by pushing, not overstepping, limits. Adrenaline surges will give the bottom an unexpected thrill, but if his or her experience is accompanied by involuntary flinching or muscular contractions, then the top can be certain that the bottom's threshold for pain has been pushed far enough and it is time to back down. If limits are overstepped (and not merely pushed), adrenaline rushes into the bloodstream, and the limbic system, overloaded with the excess charge of adrenaline and other chemical reactions to pain, causes the hypothalamus to dramatically decrease the production of dopamine. Needless to say, sexual tension will plummet! The adrenaline rush overrides the pleasure-enhancing effects of dopamine, perhaps even resulting in a self-defensive bout of aggression or anger that will most likely mark the premature end of the Sexual Ceremony. Avoid overstepping a lover's pain threshold at all costs, but note that the same intensity of contact that would cause an adrenaline rush in the above example, when provided at the height of a lengthy ceremony's blissful evolution, is likely to reveal a very different outcome: it may just push your lover over the edge into ecstasy.

The roles of tops and bottoms are elaborated upon throughout "Transcendental Techniques" and the chapter "The Joy of Play: The Roles of Provider and Receiver," but in terms of finding that dynamic balance between limits and pleasure, skilled tops are always aware of their bottoms' responses and learn to read the signs of potential sensory overload as a clear sign that it is time to lighten up, using a softer tool or shifting focus until the bottom is melting under the top's touch once again. Similarly, if a bottom seems to be becoming immune to a sensation, and the ceremony loses its pace, it is time to intensify stimulation, change the tool or technique, or move the focus from one body zone to another.

During the Sexual Ceremony, avoid causing sensory confusion by using too many different tools or practicing too many techniques at the same time. For shorter rituals that span the minimum of three hours, explore, for example, a maximum of three different techniques of full-body stimulation in combination with genital stimulation. Lovers will want to reserve their resources and avoid changing tools or techniques haphazardly. Be patient, and cater to every area of the body that can be tantalized with a tool before you put it aside. This is the most effective way to reveal the full extent of a tool's pleasure-providing capacity.

The more skilled, informed, and understanding partners become through experience, the more targeted and intentional will be the sensations that the tops provide and the more exciting and empowering will be the sensations that the bottoms receive. Once the ceremony has evolved further along its course, tops should not be surprised when truly aroused bottoms begin to beg for more direct contact than they previously agreed to explore. But unless you are journeying toward the higher dimensions of the sexual realm with an experienced partner whom you know well, always stick to the limits established before the ceremony began.

CHAPTER 12

—o—

HONOR EACH OTHER:
SAFETY

If anything is sacred, the human body is sacred.

— Walt Whitman

CONSENT, COMMUNICATE, AND CARE: when transcendental techniques are explored, these are actions that will help to ensure the positive outcome of the Paradise Found Sexual Ceremony.

PLAY FAIR

No matter how hard or soft lovers intend to play, the Sexual Ceremony evolves primarily by consent. Establish the limits of the ritual before it begins, especially if you are playing with an occasional or novice partner. While the bottom will set the boundaries of any session that entails the transcendental techniques of full-body stimulation, if either partner, the top or the bottom, does not feel perfectly comfortable, happy, and secure with the manner in which a session is progressing, that must be made known. It is a mutually shared right *and* a responsibility to interrupt the session if limits are overstepped.

Limits change, even from day to day; partners who enjoy the

effects of certain techniques may not always wish to engage in them, particularly if they feel tired or emotionally vulnerable. Similarly, partners who enjoy providing certain sensations may not always be in the mood to do so. Agreeing in advance upon the tools and techniques to be explored, before the ceremony commences, will help both partners better provide for each other's desires and wishes.

Partners must be in the spirit to play and have fun. Come into the ceremonial space both physically and mentally relaxed and prepared to transcend. Lovers must never make the mistake of coming into the ritual space with unresolved issues at heart. Failure to deal with unresolved issues before the ceremony commences is as problematic as the intentional overstepping of a bottom's boundaries. Conflict and anger have no place in the temple of erotic loving.

CHECK IN WITH YOUR PLAYMATE

Good communication skills are as fundamental to healthy relationships as they are to the positive outcome of any sexual encounter, and they become all the more relevant when using tools to explore, test, and push sexual limits. As lovers explore the potentials and powers of full-body stimulation, their desires, skills, and inevitably their sense of satisfaction will evolve through ritual after ritual.

When you play with a regular partner, do not assume that the boundaries of your last ritual will be the same the next time. What you want to explore one night may not be what you want to delve into the next. Communicating openly raises a safety net for the well-being of both partners. It reinforces their bond and allows the Sexual Ceremony to evolve harmoniously.

Partners should always feel free to guide each other physically and verbally when necessary. Whether you are topping or bottoming, if at any time you feel uncomfortable or in danger, you should interrupt the Sexual Ceremony and communicate your reason for the dissatisfaction. Make your fears as well as your needs and desires known in a way that will guarantee that they are respected—be calm, and express yourself clearly. Continue the Sexual Ceremony only if you've been able to express your concerns and you feel that they have been heard. If discomfort continues, the ritual should be brought to an end. It is a good idea to eliminate the distasteful tools or techniques from your shared repertoires if this situation occurs again with the same partner.

Skilled and respectful playmates always abide by each other's wishes and desires, and they never insist on providing sensations that have been disapproved of in the past. If your partner continues to do this, consider changing your playmate! The Sexual Ceremony should progress with respect and trust. These qualities are the foundation of any healthy relationship, and they make the difference between frustration and satisfaction, between torment and ecstasy.

Tops should "check in" with their bottoms if they are not responding positively to a given sensation, or even if they have slipped into an ecstatic, endorphin-induced trance. Checking in simply entails asking the bottom if he or she is okay and enjoying the sensations. While this practice might seem counter to that of the professional BSDM scene, being that the master or mistress of ceremonies is expected to be in total control of the situation, in the context of the Paradise Found Sexual Ceremony, it is a fundamental safety measure. Checking in will help guarantee the positive outcome of the ritual for both partners, from a physical as well as an emotional point of view.

The longer and more all encompassing a session grows, the more important the simple act of checking in becomes. In extended sessions, both partners are likely to experience trancelike states from the emission of the theta brain-wave frequency and endorphin and hormone elation. But the top must never forget to remain aware of the bottom's psychophysiological state and be ready to respond accordingly.

CARE FOR YOUR PARTNER

Pushing sexual limits within a controlled and well-organized ritual environment over extended periods of arousal has the power not only to elevate the practitioners to transcendental degrees of sexual satisfaction but also to unveil the core of the inner spirit. Extensive and particularly intense periods of stimulation may lead to the rare and unexpected release of deep, formerly unconscious emotions. This emotional symphony, known as catharsis, is instigated through the overstimulation of the limbic system. The complex functions and structures of this enigmatic part of the brain are still cause for academic dispute, but most researchers agree that the interrelated structures of the limbic system allow us to perceive pleasure as well as pain. Associated with self-preservation and instincts, the limbic system is associated with our innate drive to seek the principal motivators of life—pleasure and happiness.

One of the limbic system's key glands is the hypothalamus. The hypothalamus not only secretes hormones and synthesizes endorphins but also serves as a link, via the pituitary gland, to both the nervous system and the endocrine system. The hypothalamus is one of the glands that produce the hormone dopamine, which also acts as a neurotransmitter; its production induces a "drifty" sense of happiness and serenity. Playtime, no matter our age or the activities we are enjoying, also stimulates another complex zone of the limbic system known as the hippocampus. Among other functions, this paleomammalian area of the cerebral cortex is associated with the input, storage, and output of memories. The amygdala, another important part of the limbic system, coordinates behavioral responses to emotional stimuli, including those emotions provoked by pleasure and pain as well as by memories. The fact that our responses to pleasure and pain are in grand part processed by same area of the brain—the limbic system—helps explain why the line between pleasure and pain is so fine, as well as why sensations that would be painful if administered outside of a sexual context can also be excruciatingly blissful.

Like all deeply emotional forms of release, catharsis can evoke tears. If your ceremony brings this emotional release to the surface, stay calm, embrace the moment, and treat your own, or your partner's, reactions with care. A healthy cry can dissolve barriers and leave one feeling liberated, if not spiritually purified. The more you care about your partner, the easier it will be to deal with the eventuality of catharsis. When the tears are dried, you will both feel happier and healthier.

As your playtimes become more evolved and sophisticated, you will find yourself curious about pushing your sexual limits. More intense sensations and heightened psychological impact may be attained through the use of any given tool or technique, but then skill, knowledge, and safety become increasingly relevant.

"Safe" words should be implemented when the bottom's limits are being tested or pushed. In a ceremony that involves more extreme techniques, stronger sensations, or any form of play in which the bottom may need or want to quickly inform a top of his or her needs, the safe word makes for an "out." The most common safe words are colors, because they are easy to remember. Saying "yellow" can mean, "Slow down. This is getting too intense." Calling out "blue" can indicate, "I have had enough of what you are doing. Please stop." Crying out "red," can mean "Stop everything. You have surpassed my limits!" If a top surpasses the bottom's limits to the degree that the bottom must voice the safe word "red," the session should definitely come to an end.

Progressing gradually toward more intense sensations and alternating between these and subtler, less direct forms of stimulation will help avoid the use of safe words as well as ensure extended periods of transcendental playtime.

SUBMIT TO THE EXPERIENCE

Naturally, the most direct way to become experienced with any tool or technique is to submit to the skilled hand of the ceremonial partner. If you find yourself in the adventurous hands of a partner who has yet to be initiated in the use of any given tool or technique, it is up to you, the person on the receiving end, to guide your novice top. Once you are experienced in that tool or technique, and you are eager to submit to it, invite the novice to submit first to you. You will need to emphasize not only the *do*s but also the *do not*s.

In the case that both partners are novices to the powers of a tool, they may decide to take turns, either administering or submitting to the new sensations. This experience will prevent a top from underestimating the potency of any tool he or she may choose to wield. Experiencing a tool's power personally is essential to mastering its use.

A lover who refuses to submit, even once, to a tool that he or she intends to use on another will not be fully aware of the tool's assets or limits. When you are not at all keen on a new sensation in question, request that the bottom try the tool on himself or herself, before proceeding. When new tools and techniques are incorporated into your playtime, their powers and potentials should be unveiled gradually. Savor the sense of discovery that exploring the unknown holds, and adjust to the new experiences at your own pace. Do not set sexual goals, as your sexual journey will unfold naturally with practice. It is through practice that we expand our sensual repertoires, hurdle limits, refine sexual skills, and reap heightened sexual satisfaction.

A FINAL WORD ON HONORING EACH OTHER

· Taking a general first-aid class is important, whether you play hard or not. It prepares for the eventuality of any emergency, even beyond the boudoir.

. If you suffer or who have suffered from medical conditions, particularly a heart condition, speak to your doctor about the risk of submitting to the more invigorating forms of play, like erotic flagellation or movement restraint. If you are under the impression that your doctor is not open-minded, seek out a alternative sex-friendly medical expert. You may even invite him or her to read the chapters of *The Boudoir Bible* related to your interests; it will speed up the process. Establishing an open and honest relationship with your doctor is important.

. View your implements of desire as sacred objects. They are only intended for use by adults, so keep them out of the sight and reach of children. If used by those who are unaware of their power, certain tools can inflict undesirable harm.

. If you are traveling by air and you don't want to leave home without a few of your favorite instruments, pack them carefully inside your checked baggage, as long as they are not intrinsically valuable. This will avoid potential embarrassment from custom officials or at airport security sites.

Let us now prepare to transcend!

CHAPTER 13

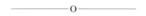

THE TOUCH OF A FEATHER:
EROTIC TICKLING

Invest in a feather duster—the possibilities are endless.

— Anne Rice

EROTIC TICKLING IS one of the simplest yet most versatile techniques of full-body stimulation. At the beginning of the Sexual Ceremony, tickling opens the sensory channels; during a lengthy Sexual ceremony, erotic tickling can recharge the sexual energy of a seemingly satiated lover (who may have slipped into an ecstatic slumber) and jump-start another round of Paradise Found. It is also a very sweet way to bring an intense ritual to a lingering end. Erotic tickling can be performed during peaking to divert an over-aroused partner's attention from the genitals, slowing the rhythm of the ceremony. But it can quicken its pace as well. Its capacity to guide a receptive partner from one psychophysiological dimension to another with ease is one of its greatest merits.

Some people have a real aversion to tickling and cannot help curling into a defensive fetal position at even the slightest feathery touch. Those who respond negatively to erotic tickling may be making an unconscious association with a less-than-joyful childhood tickle session: being tickle-tortured by siblings or peers to the point of ultimate humiliation—wet underwear!

While it is true that some partners may like to push the fine line between pleasure and torture and laughter makes us feel good with its surge of antidepressant, muscle-relaxing endorphins, hysterical bouts of laughter are not the aim in the erotic context. When tickling is performed skillfully, satisfied partners may emit a pleasurable giggle from time to time or sigh contentedly, but if they happen to break out in nervous or hysterical laughter, this reaction probably indicates that the sensations are less than erotic.

TITILLATING TICKLE TOOLS

The body is naturally equipped with some very efficient ticklers, from the slightest touch of the soft, padded tips of the fingers to the tongue's rousing energy. In German, the clitoris is called the *kitzler*, which means a tickler—and the clitoris responds to a tickle like no other part of the body! Women may use their nipples to simultaneously tickle a lover and stimulate themselves. Long hair, as well, is an excellent tickling tool.

Lovers may choose from a variety of instruments for tickling. Feathers have an aesthetic appeal besides having the ability to elicit a thrilling variety of sensations. Using two (possibly different) feathers, one in each hand, will double the sensorial impact. The classic ostrich feather is soft, fluffy, and wide enough to caress large areas of the body. Imagine the delights of an ostrich feather fan!

Ostrich feathers are also long, so they allow the purveyor of pleasure, the top, to have a bit of distance from the bottom. Distance permits the top to better observe the bottom's reactions as well as enhancing eye contact between partners, which reinforces the pleasure bond. Long pheasant feathers give a similar distance, but they tend to be pricklier. Glossy black cock feathers have a similarly sensuous appeal, but they are medium in length. Marabou stork feathers, on the other hand, are short, extremely soft, and particularly suited for close-contact tickling. Feather dusters can make for fabulous tickling tools. (Make certain they are reserved for this purpose alone!). Classic "French maid" models with wooden handles can be found in the housewares section of many stores.

Silks, scarves, fur, and a lanky horsetail whip can also be used to transform the entire body into a sensual, sexually receptive organ. Soft paintbrushes from Asian-themed gift shops or art supply stores can be used to paint your lover wild with passion. Those made of soft white horsehair, mounted on beautiful bamboo or lacquered wooden handles, are more aesthetically appealing than paintbrushes from a hardware store, permitting them to be taken out of their home-improvement context and incorporated into the Sexual Ceremony with greater conviction. Use your imagination! Virtually anything of a subtle, feathery nature may be used to tickle.

In fact, even potentially more extreme tools such as leather whips, crops, and floggers (described in the chapter "X Marks the Spot: Erotic Flagellation") can be used for ethereal, indirect caresses. Whenever one of these stricter tools is used for direct and intense impact, the receiver should also be given softer, sweeter sensations as well. This not only avoids predictability by fostering the thrill of anticipation but reminds the bottom that his or her top really does care.

The brain functions in such a way that it's nearly impossible to tickle yourself. But during a solo masturbation ritual, try softly brushing yourself with feathers, fur, and the like; you may find that you can trick the brain. Those who feel an aversion to erotic tickling are encouraged to reevaluate its power through this method.

If your partner is not completely convinced but consents to your erotic tickling whims all the same, do not attempt to provide these subtle sensations until he or she is fully sexually aroused. If your partner is tense, offer an erotic massage; engage in other forms of erotic play you know are enjoyed. When your lover is truly relaxed and receptive, erotic tickling can even take the place of a preparatory massage.

LIMITLESS RAPTURE

When it comes to tickling, there are no "no" zones, but in order to provide erotic pleasure and incite pure joy, tickle the areas of the body that are less sensitive before those that are more sensitive to touch. Generally, less sensitive zones of the body are those regularly exposed to the elements or that present more muscle mass or where hair grows more readily. The upper back, the base of the neck, and the outer surfaces of the upper and lower arms are a few good places to commence a tickle ritual.

Once those areas have been sensitized, the lower back, the crooks of the knees, the backs of the thighs, and the buttocks may be approached with the slight touch. The buttocks are more erotically charged than the back, especially on the sweet spot—the area where the buttocks connect with the legs (see plate XIV, page 222). Alternately tickling these areas and the less sensitive areas of the body will build tension gradually; it may also aid even the most adamant of anti-ticklers to ease into the pleasures of this delightfully subtle contact.

The even more sensitive areas of the body, where blood vessels and nerve endings lie closer to the surface of the skin, are next: the neck, the armpits, the inner arms, the sides of the breasts and the torso, the ribs, the palms of the hands, the inner thighs, the crooks of the elbows, the fine skin of the ankles and the wrists, and finally the inner soles of the feet and the areas between the toes. Here erotic tickling will make a vivid impact.

Most lovers must be highly sexually aroused in order to perceive the erogenous capacity of these fine-skinned areas, whose power to heighten one's sense of sexual satisfaction often goes under-evaluated, forgotten, or ignored during PGO sex. Within a Sexual Ceremony, however, lovers have the time to explore them. Stimulating these areas can gauge a lover's readiness, push his or her limits, or serve as a key to opening the doors to Paradise over and over again.

WORSHIP EVERY INCH OF YOUR LOVER'S BODY

If you have tested your partner's receptivity to subtle degrees of contact, and you have managed to coax them into a receptive state, you might invite him or her to submit to a full-fledged tickle ritual. Ask your partner to roll over onto his or her back and spread his or her legs and arms ever so slightly. This position will provide easy access to all of the most sensitive erogenous zones of the body. Once your lover is comfortable, you might begin with a deep, long explorative kiss, then proceed to tantalize the ears, eyelids, and the neck, including the nape where the hairline begins, with the slightest of caresses from feathers, fur, or your lips and tongue. Then begin a gradual descent. (If you yearn to *be* tickled, take this as a guide to the possibilities of your pleasure!)

Erotic tickling has the advantage of being one of the most pleasurably effective means to map out the sensory landscape of your lover's body, from head to toe. The intimate information can be used to a positive end in this and every other Sexual Ceremony with the same partner, no matter what tool or technique is being explored. For example, if your lover's skin prickles with pleasure while you are caressing the sides of her breasts with a feathery touch; if he writhes or moans uncontrollably while you tantalize his ears or neck; if she loses all sense of control when you tickle her inner thighs or tug her hair, make a mental note of these responses. Tickling reveals the highly charged erogenous zones of a lover's body, as well as those areas that provoke a less than positive response.

For example, take into consideration one highly sensitive area: the feet. Some love to have their feet tickled, kissed, and sucked, while others will cringe and recoil with nervous tension at the sight of a feather quivering over apprehensively curled toes! When you approach your lover's feet, and his or her response to your attention is anything but positive, that limit should be respected. That said, it would be a mistake to completely eliminate the feet from your ceremonial explorations! Over time, with practice and experience, our needs and desires change and evolve, as does our relationship with our bodies. Over the course of elaborating the Sexual Ceremony, you may likely appreciate sensations that previously you had judged unpleasant or unacceptable. Parts of the body that had been off-limits may come to reveal themselves as golden keys to the transcendental realm of the ecstatic dimension.

During the tickle ritual, as with any other form of extra-genital stimulation during the Sexual Ceremony, the genitals will be a point of return. Not only are the genitals the primary source of the sexual vibration, but they are the most delightfully vulnerable and sensitive flesh of the entire body.

Try working from the center of the body outward. Stroke, suck, lick, and venerate your lover's genitals, then move toward the less obvious erogenous zones. Gradually stimulate one area of his or her yearning body, then another, with the slightest of loving caresses. Watch your lover's skin prickle with goose bumps, then move your intention back toward the center of the body. Tease by tickling the areas surrounding the genitals before rewarding them with more direct contact.

Establish a steady, intimate rhythm using your body's tools (fingers, tongue, lips, nipples, hair, and more) in combination with feathers, fur, and any other tool of your choice to entice your lover into an electric pleasure dance. From time to time, draw back and make him or her anticipate your touch. This will build excitement and send your lover into a sexy, libidinous spin. Alternate between genital and extra-genital contact as well as subtle and more intense degrees of sensation. This avoids predictability and reinforces the physical and the psychological impact of the ritual as well. Gradually pushing the bottom's sensory limits prompts a surge in the production of endorphins.

Worship every inch of your lover's body with the sole intent to please; bring sexual tension to the heights, and you'll have him or her begging for more. Each time the tickle tool diverts your lover's focus from his or her genitals toward other erogenous zones, visualize the sexual energy spreading throughout your partner's body, and invite him or her to do the same. As the ceremony progresses, his or her perception of each subsequent caress becomes enhanced, and sexual tension escalates. And each time you, the purveyor of sensations, return to worship your lover's genitals, they'll be further charged with ecstatic energy. When performed skillfully, erotic tickling, like any other technique of full-body stimulation, will provide great pleasure as well as instill intense levels of concentration that can result in trancelike states in both partners. (But note that if your ceremonial partner is a man, the softest touch of your feather, in combination with direct genital contact, may catapult him straight into the wild haze of orgasm. Postpone this end of the ceremony by immediately diverting your—and his— attention from his genitals to other, less sensitive areas of the body until he regains control.)

As erotic tickling is a very subtle form of full-body stimulation, the provider of sensations must prevent the ritual from losing its edge. If you are on the receiving end, and your top doesn't seem to notice you are no longer responding ecstatically, tell him or her what you need! Tops, if your bottom seems immune to the charms of tickling, focus on more sensitive areas of the body, or provide more direct sensations to ensure the ceremony's transcendental progression.

THRILLING CHILLS: LOVE BITES AND CAT SCRATCHES

Delectable love bites and careful yet passionate cat scratches can be used to test a bottom's growing receptivity and send thrilling chills up and down the spine. If these forms of stimulation incite a positive response, the top may be assured that more intense forms of stimulation than tickling will be appreciated.

Your lover may enjoy having his or her feet, head, back, or buttocks carefully bitten and scratched. Other areas of the body that may be bitten as well as scratched include the shoulders, the upper arms, and the backs of the legs. The neck will also respond vividly to careful love bites. The sensitive skin of the penis, when erect, and the scrotum, when tightened, can be carefully scratched to delight. Avoid biting these areas, however, unless your lover requests such attention.

Keep in mind that while long fingernails may be effective in erotic tickling and scratching, they are not well adapted to other forms of hand-to-body contact, particularly when the female genitals or the anus of either sex is involved. (Keeping the nails on both the fingers and the toes short not only avoids having lovers unintentionally injure each other, it also broadens the range of sensations that can be provided manually.) With a little bit of imagination, a myriad of alternatives to long fingernails can be found. While classic backscratchers that terminate with miniature hands are an effective and obvious solution, take the time to poke around in antique boutiques and Asian-themed gift shops for other exquisite possibilities. Miniature appetizer forks in sterling silver and bamboo, vintage cocktail ornaments, wooden hair ornaments, and decorative combs can all find a new and decidedly more ecstatic purpose in the boudoir. A little research will lead to the discovery of a variety of aesthetic sources of erotic scratching.

No matter which instrument you choose, make sure that it is

not too sharp or pointed. Test the object on your own forearm before putting it into ceremonial action on your partner's skin. Unlike tickling, which elicits a rosy color, scratching and love biting can leave very distinct marks that may take anywhere from an hour to a few days to disappear. Since leaving marks on a lover's body is not always appropriate, it's best to establish this limit before the ceremony commences. Some lovers enjoy being marked and consider the traces of a passionate round of Paradise Found souvenirs of ecstasy. In the case that your attentions have left undesired marks, soothe them with an ice pack. If the skin is chafed or scratched, apply an antiseptic cream.

One of the greatest benefits of experimenting in the ritualized context is that coming to appreciate new sensations broadens sexual horizons. Even the most adamant of anti-ticklers has been known to convert to the powers of the feather. Once a top has skillfully mapped out the bottom's sensory landscape, the shared act will have unveiled physical limits as well as the "hot" spots. Taking "the long way around" in the sensual journey will lead you both straight to Paradise.

CHAPTER 14

———— o ————

PUSHING THE THRESHOLD:
CLAMPS

Endure and persist; this pain will turn to good by and by.

— Ovid

HIGHLY SENSITIVE SURFACES of the body such as the nipples, the shaft of the penis, and the labia majora respond vividly to intense sensations. These small areas of flesh can be carefully constricted with the fingertips or with clamps to call upon the erotic powers of the endorphin rush.

Making love prompts the production of oxytocin, but nipple stimulation and nipple constriction will cause this potent natural antidepressant to surge into the bloodstream. Scientific research has revealed that this hormone, also released during orgasm, plays a fundamental role in sexual bonding, so to encourage its flow with erotic intent not only feels good but also reinforces the intimate bond with your partner.

Women's nipples are connected directly to the genitals by the nervous system and "light up" the pleasure centers in the brain in much the same way genital stimulation does—it is for this reason that some women can actually orgasm from their stimulation. Women's nipples become even more sensitive during ovulation, and their sensitivity gradually decreases with the onset of the monthly cycle.

While male nipples are considered to be less sensitive than female nipples, some men find their stimulation extremely arousing. Male or female, constricting the erectile tissue that forms the nipples will incite an endorphin rush.

ON THE EDGE

Lovers who enjoy having their nipples pinched and pulled are likely to enjoy the more intense degrees of sensation that clamps can provide. The fact that they leave the hands of the pleasure provider free to roam is one advantage of these little tools. Clamps are commonly associated with BDSM "edge play," erotic-play practices that push one's threshold for pain. But the pain or pleasure will vary according to the device's design.

Mind you, there are clamps, and there are *CLAMPS*! One should never be fooled by appearances; even the daintiest of these devices can make a *big* sensory impact. Nipple clamps come in many shapes and sizes and provide anywhere from moderate to extreme sensations, depending on the degree of constriction they cause and the quantity of flesh they seize. In some cases, the smaller the bite, the meaner they are!

Like most of the instruments that stimulate the body beyond the genitals, nipple clamps are now readily available online. But rarely if ever do they arrive in the mailboxes of adventurous patrons with instructions for their safe use. Yet in order to incite the most positive response and avoid injury, lovers must follow certain guidelines when using nipple clamps.

Nipple clamps, like any implement of desire designed for more intense stimulation, should be used only in the context of extended playtime. Leave them on the altar or bedside table until your lover, who has already consented to the use of their constrictive grip to push the limit between pleasure and pain, is truly well aroused. Otherwise, he or she may be unable to withstand their initial, intense impact.

If you are a novice to the power of the clamp, or you do not wish to make the investment, wooden clothespins (the kind with metal springs) make an excellent alternative and are a good introduction to the powers of constriction. Do not use clothespins made of plastic, however; these can damage the skin and are less aesthetically pleasing. Unless your lover enjoys intense degrees of constriction, use the standard size. As adorable as they are, the miniature variety can be more aggressive than the standard clothespin, as they pinch smaller areas of flesh.

No matter what you decide to use—a wooden clothespin or clamps designed specifically for the purpose of erotic nipple constriction—test the grip on yourself before trying them on your lover. The webbed area of the hand between the thumb and forefinger is suitable for experimenting, although the best way to get an accurate impression of a clamp's sensory impact is to test it on erectile tissue. If this is not an option, clasp one onto your lower lip; also composed of erectile tissue, it can provide you with a realistic impression of the clamp's potential.

WRITHING UNDER THE INFLUENCE

To put nipple clamps in place, tantalize one of your well-aroused lover's nipples to attention; then, holding its tender flesh between the tips of your thumb and forefinger, pull it gently away from his or her body. Carefully place the clamp at the base of the nipple—not on the tip! The less flesh you take into the clamp's grip, the more likely it is to cause sensations that will be interpreted as painful and unbearably nonerotic. If the clamp is placed correctly, what is perceived initially as discomfort will, by the time the second clamp has been put into place (thanks to the analgesic surge of endorphins), gradually become muted into a deeply arousing rush of intense sensation. As your lover writhes under the influence of the clamps, distract his or her attention from the now highly sensitized nipples by coaxing the sexual vibration to flow throughout his or her entire being with a shower of sweet sensations—kiss, stroke, make love to your lover, and he or she will soar.

But even in the midst of ecstasy, you and your partner need to remain aware of the duration of time that the nipple is being clamped. The greatest mistake that lovers can make is to leave nipple clamps in place for too long. A clamped partner may well be able to tolerate a relatively high level of pain-cum-pleasure, but clamps should never be left in place for more than fifteen minutes at a time. Keeping tight clamps in place longer may injure the delicate erectile tissues of the nipples and even damage the nerve endings, permanently reducing the nipples' sensitivity.

Avoid getting so wrapped up in the fun that you forget that the clamps are in place! A lover flying high on the wings of the body's natural love drug is transcending the boundaries of the physical; thus, it is the responsibility of the partner providing sensations to remove the clamps at the right time. The use of clamps demands that the top be highly in tune with the bottom at all times. Endorphins make us feel good and increase our tolerance for pain, but they also reduce our capacity to make clear, quick decisions.

The removal of clamps from highly sensitized nipples should be done lovingly and carefully. Once the clamp has been taken off, encourage the free flow of blood circulation back into the area with the slightest tickles, the sweetest licks, and the softest of caresses.

Some clamps are designed for use on the nipples alone. Others can also be applied to the scrotum, the shaft of the penis, or the outer lips of the vulva. For a thrill, try applying wooden clothespins on less sensitive areas of your lover's body—for example, apply anywhere from ten to twenty clothespins to the fleshy areas of the back or along the spinal column. Once they are in place, strum them with your fingertips until it is time to remove them, and then do so slowly, one by one. To enhance the dynamics of the ritual, remove the clamps with the perfect aim and accurate flick of a crop's leather tip. (Note that this method should never be used to remove clamps from the genitals or the nipples.)

When the clamps are removed, circulation will rush back into each area that was constricted, their release inciting yet another surge of endorphins in a revitalizing charge. As the Sexual Ceremony progresses, the clamps may be reapplied, but only if the receiving partner acquiesces. Some will prefer that the places that have been clamped be avoided altogether after they have been sensitized to this degree—especially the tender nipples. Safety guidelines do not exclude the receiver of such intoxicating sensations from reciprocating. Via the same constrictive route, lovers can unite on a lofty plateau in Paradise!

CHAPTER 15

———o———

SOME LIKE IT HOT:
TEMPERATURE PLAY

The only abnormality is the incapacity to love.

— Anaïs Nin

TEMPERATURE PLAY can be a surprisingly effective and dramatically sensual way to charge an aroused lover with sexual vibrations. Hot wax and ice can sensitize areas of the body with tingly heat or thrilling chills. The psychophysiological charge of temperature play can spill endorphins into the system, making for an exhilarating and effective prelude to more intense and direct forms of stimulation.

RED-HOT ADVENTURES

Hot wax is potentially unpredictable and even dangerous, so use common sense to ensure that your ritual endeavors result in ecstasy, not agony! The candles that create the aura of your temple should not be employed for hot wax play unless they are made with pure paraffin, which is used often in church lights and kosher candles. Pure paraffin melts between 117°F and 147°F (47°C and 64°C), while beeswax and the wax of common colored and perfumed candles melt at higher temperatures. Candles other than paraffin are therefore not safe for hot wax play, even in the case of partners who like to sharpen the edge of their sensory limits. Hot wax play should provide for intensely pleasant sensations, not burns!

Hot wax play was once categorized as BDSM edge play, but massage or lotion candles made of soy, cocoa butter, coconut oil, vitamin E, and other natural, skin-nurturing substances have taken the algolagnist edge out of the technique. Available through most erotica suppliers, particularly those dedicated primarily to women, the wax of these specially made candles melts at a much lower temperature than paraffin, eliminating the risk of burns. The hot oil that drips from these candles does not harden as it cools—it is to be rubbed into a lucky lover's skin. Massage candles are a sensuous introduction to traditional hot wax play.

Molten wax cools as it falls, so before dripping hot wax onto a lover's skin, calculate the approximate distance from which the candle should be held from the body by dripping some wax onto your own forearm. Traditional candles would need to be held at a much higher distance from the body than massage candles. If you are using candles made of paraffin, rub some mineral oil onto the skin first to facilitate the removal of the wax.

Wax is likely to land with a splash, so protect the area where you will be playing with a bedsheet, a towel, or a latex sheet. Once you are done, simply roll it up and put it aside—the ceremony should not be interrupted by either of you feeling obliged to clean up while the ritual is in progress! (As bedsheets or towels may need to be disposed of or sent to the cleaners after such use, an eco-friendly alternative is a latex sheet; not only will wax not adhere to its surface, but a latex sheet is easy to clean and reusable.)

The more obvious erogenous zones of the body will respond vividly to hot wax play. Essentially any area below the neckline can be sensitized through hot wax application. The breasts and nipples respond well to these sensations, just as the genitals do—as long as they are fully depilated, or as long as those areas with hair are avoided. (Pulling wax from hair is guaranteed to push the limits between pleasure and pain just a little too far for some.) Those who wish to integrate depilation into the Sexual Ceremony's elaboration should use cosmetic wax; it is designed specifically for that purpose.

Before commencing hot wax play, tops must make certain that the bottom is relaxed, well aroused, and receptive to the idea. If sensitive areas are approached gradually, the power of anticipation will further the overall impact of the session. Novices appreciate a preview of the sensations on the less-sensitive areas of the back, until they feel completely comfortable with the hot wax application.

Some lovers consider wax removal as much fun as its application. If large surfaces of the body have been sensitized, the bottom will need to shower and scrub down to remove every trace of wax from their skin. When serious coverage is the plan, you may wish to practice hot wax play prior to an intermission or at the end of the Sexual Ceremony. Lovers must respect the fact that not everyone is ready to explore, test, or push sensory limits, so progress gradually, with a sense of adventure, not obligation.

ICE-COLD EXPLOITS

Stimulating the surface of a well-aroused lover's warm skin with an ice cube will incite psychophysiological reactions similar to the intense sensations of hot wax. In fact, if both ice and hot wax are used in alternation, the session's evolution will be all the more moving. Ice can be used to tantalize any part of the body, including those areas with body hair. Above the neckline, however, the lips and mouth are the only zones that will respond positively to being seductively tortured with a chill. Ice will call the nipples to immediate attention, but it is likely to have the opposite effect on an erect penis or clitoris, unless the application is fleeting! This curbing power of ice can be put to creative use while a man is peaking. Like the penis, the clitoris will also respond well to being stimulated with ice in alternation with any other sensation that will warm it right back up again. Once the chill subsides, blood will rush into and invigorate the area, which will crave the reward of further contact.

Popping an ice cube into your mouth during oral stimulation will turn the sexual tension in an over-aroused male lover down a notch or two, but once the ice has melted, be prepared to handle the added increment of bliss; his skin will be twice as sensitive to your warm touch. Inserting a cube of ice into the vagina (as long as it has been sucked first to soften its edges) will also give a chilling thrill. On the other hand, slipping ice inside the anus is likely to cause uncomfortable cramping.

On a sweltering summer's day, an ice massage becomes a soothing preliminary, intermission, or conclusion to the Sexual Ceremony. Fill a large bowl with ice, cover it with cold water, and toss in a small hand towel. Invite your lover to lie down, and use the cold, wet towel to rub his or her entire body, from head to toe. Wipe away excess water with a dry towel as you proceed. The icy massage will send blood rushing to the surface of the skin and leave your lover feeling invigorated and ready to warm things up again.

There are many other ways to bring temperature play, to the temple. Use your imagination—beware of red-hot peperoncini, but don't ignore the erotic potential of seemingly innocent breath mints, herbal-based heat rubs, and mentholated ointments, and even a cup of hot tea. *Au plaisir!*

CHAPTER 16

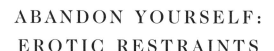

ABANDON YOURSELF:
EROTIC RESTRAINTS

The deepest feeling always shows itself in silence; not in silence,
but restraint.

— Marianne Moore, "Silence"

CATERING TO any one sense heightens the capacity of the other senses, which augments the perception of pleasure. But as paradoxical as it may seem, temporary sensory deprivation is also a powerful erotic enhancement—in particular, the techniques for restraining the senses of sight, hearing, and movement. These techniques charge the limbic system, ignite the flames of desire, and lead lovers to abandon themselves to pleasure and experience entirely different pinnacles of sexual arousal and satisfaction.

You may wonder why I consider movement a sense. During the past fifty years, scientific research in sensory perception has added to Aristotle's limited definition of a mere five senses. According to some physiologists, human beings have twenty perceptual functions, if not more. These include thermoception, the perception of hot or cold; equilibrioception, the perception of balance; proprioception, the perception of body awareness; and nociception, the perception of pain. (Oddly enough, I have searched for but have yet to stumble across the neurological term for the perception of pleasure. If you are in the know, please do share.) The perception of movement is considered by modern scientists to be "the sixth sense." Though this term is most commonly associated with the paranormal, phenomena such as telepathy or clairvoyance are better described as *extra*sensory perception.

Over the past fifty years, neurophysiologists have contributed enormously to our understanding of the wildly enigmatic senses and the still deeply misunderstood perceptive capacity of the brain. The effects of sensory deprivation on the human mind and body were the focus of Dr. John C. Lilly, who, in 1954, in order to study these effects, invented the sensory deprivation tank, now also called the flotation, REST, or isolation tank. (His conclusions helped me understand why the temporary loss of sight, hearing, and movement can make such a positive impact on lovers' sexual satisfaction—read on to find out.)

The flotation tank is an enclosed, soundproof tub containing mineral water and large doses of Epsom salts. Once the subject settles comfortably into the water, the tank is closed, completely isolating the subject from external stimuli. The high concentration of salt in the water, which is maintained at body temperature, causes the subject to float. As soon as the subject begins to relax into and adjust to the effects of total and complete sensory isolation, his or her brain ceases to generate the beta and alpha brain-wave frequencies inherent to normal waking consciousness and begins to generate the theta brain-wave frequency. Subjects describe the experience as transcendental, otherworldly, deeply meditative, and rejuvenating—the boundaries of the physical body are said to seem to dissolve, accompanied by an overall sense of well-being.

Restraining a lover's sense of sight, hearing, movement, or all three at once, prompts similar results in the context of the Sexual Ceremony. The techniques of erotic restraint incite the emission of alpha brain waves, whose deep, calming effects oblige the bottom to "drop in" to a sexually receptive state of mind and body almost instantly, allowing him or her to focus keenly on the sensations. It also forces the senses that are not being restrained to compensate, becoming more acute—as does the lover's perception of pleasure, which is in turn then reinforced by the emission of the transcendental theta brain-wave frequency.

By the 1970s, the flotation tank had been adopted by various schools of alternative medicine for its healing powers, to counteract the effects of stress, pain, insomnia, and anxiety. Continued research in sensory deprivation revealed that the deliberate removal of stimuli from the senses strokes the pleasure centers of the brain, increasing the production of analgesic endorphins and hormones. And the positive effects of these chemicals in combination with the theta brain-wave frequency has been expounded on throughout *The Boudoir Bible*!

SEXUAL SURRENDER

The tools and techniques of erotic restraint crystallize the roles of the bottom and the top, which have been described in the chapter "The Joy of Play: The Roles of Provider and Receiver." The bottom is essentially obliged to surrender the control of his or her pleasure to the top. This power shift creates an intense psychophysiological charge that reinforces the sexual bond like no other transcendental technique. Erotic restraint of sight and movement are also known to have the power to dissolve latent sexual inhibitions. The techniques have even been reported to heal both anorgasmia in women and impotency in men—yes, when practiced with consent and skill between trusting partners, erotic restraint is really that good! It helps lovers to "drop in" to a sexually receptive state of mind and body almost instantly and incites acute perceptual awareness, prompting ever more wanton states of sexual arousal and an endorphin high.

But fear of abandoning one's self to pleasure and losing control, despite it being essential to experiencing deep sexual satisfaction, keeps many lovers from exploring the ecstatic potential of erotic restraint. It is understandable, on the surface, that even a slight degree of sensory restraint—a corset, blindfold, or handcuff, for example—is considered by most as an infringement on one's personal will and freedom. After all, only fifty years have passed since most Westerners, whatever their gender or sexual orientation, have had the privilege to be able to choose how and with whom they might express their sexuality. Women, in particular, may view the use of erotic restraints as a step backward for female empowerment and an affirmation of outmoded male superiority. But erotic restraint is actually a generous invitation to please and to be pleased. To consent to such bliss is, in actuality, a way of saying, "I trust you."

It must be understood that when lovers *choose* to practice erotic restraint, they are neither victims nor perpetrators of sexual violence or abuse but, instead, adventurous and trusting sexual accomplices. Lovers who appreciate its effects (whether they categorize themselves as BDSM or not) do not necessarily seek or need pain in order to be sexually satisfied. In fact, the tools of erotic restraint should restrict the senses, not inflict pain; if they do, the bottom will be distracted all too soon from the real goal of the session—deep pleasure. Just as the top must remain attentive at all times to the bottom's comfort, it is the bottom's responsibility to alert his or her top immediately if there is unwanted pain, making those feelings known either verbally or through signs or safe words agreed upon in advance. (The use of these and other safety essentials are outlined in the chapter "Honor Each Other: Safety," which is an essential read before engaging in any form of limit-pushing sexual techniques.)

The bottom should call for an intermission to the session if the discomfort cannot be resolved by the top through slight modifications to the degree of restraint or in the bottom's position. Erotic sensory deprivation requires unequivocal trust between partners; as a top *or* bottom, if you do not know your chosen partner well and have yet to establish this degree of confidence in each other, refrain from using the tools and techniques of erotic restraint until you do.

A DELECTABLE PRIVILEGE: PLAY RESPONSIBLY

The restraint of movement, sight, or hearing can be introduced at any moment during the evolution of a Sexual Ceremony and practiced in combination with genital and extra-genital stimulation. Note that some lovers find the deprivation of more than one sense at a time too intense, while others live for combined sensory deprivation! Experimentation is the only way to test, reveal, and stretch your limits. Once the bottom has been restrained, the role of the top is to guide him or her toward an exhilarating, full-bodied sexual experience and ultimately coax the bottom to transcend the earthly barriers of body, time, and space in ecstasy.

As with all of the transcendental techniques that we have explored, it is the bottom who primarily establishes the limits of the session. His or her desire to explore the sexual dimension via a form of erotic restraint should be interpreted as a sign of great trust to be honored by the top, who is granted the delectable privilege of administering such pleasures. The role of a restrained bottom is to enjoy and surrender to the top's generous intentions. This does not imply that the bottom is passive, however. On the contrary, a bottom is highly in tune with and responsive to his or her top. Even though some forms of movement restraint prevent the bottom from being able to make manual contact with the top, the most mutually empowering positions will allow the top to receive oral stimulation or the pleasures of penetration. If the bottom is not orally restrained, verbal feedback may also serve to stimulate the top.

For the top, providing physical pleasure by establishing a steady, uninterrupted crescendo of sensations is the primary objective, but he or she is equally responsible for the bottom's well-being, as the restrained bottom is physically and emotionally sensitive and vulnerable. As the top introduces tools and techniques, he or she must do so with loving care and skillful control. The more skillful and creative the top is in orchestrating the session's rhythm, the more likely both partners will be to experience the meditative trance-like states that are inherent to erotic restraint, and the more probable it is that the bottom will transcend!

It is also the top's responsibility, before the implementation of any form of restraint, to make sure that all of the necessary tools are organized and at hand's reach. The reason for this is that once the ceremony commences, the top should not abandon the restrained bottom for any reason. To leave a restrained bottom alone, even if the bottom is able to set himself or herself free with little effort, is not recommended. During the practice of visual restraint and more extreme forms of movement restraint, emergencies may arise that will require the top's presence to address. If it is part of the session to "abandon" the restrained bottom, this must be done with fore-thought and extreme care. Ritual abandonment can certainly be staged to incite a desired emotional response, but remember that the reenactment is not real—one does not actually leave the temple.

In order to evolve harmoniously, erotic restraint sessions must be organized in advance. Setting out all of the tools at hand's reach will ensure that the top remains in close physical contact with the bottom at all times, giving the bottom a sense of security and facilitating the top's ability to provide an uninterrupted ascent to Paradise. Even a flashlight should be set out—no one can predict an electrical blackout! Flashlights can also be used to get a better view of your intimate activities (of course, only as long as the bottom enjoys a little loving humiliation or intimate exposure). Comfortable cushions and a couple of warm, soft blankets might also come in handy during the session and will definitely be appreciated once the bottom is released. A bottle of water should also be opened and a straw provided for the bottom's easy sipping.

Another responsibility of the top is to verify the bottom's overall satisfaction and well-being. (The happy bottom must also remember to check in with himself or herself throughout the session.) The sound of the top's voice in the bottom's ears, just like the touch of the top's hands, brings a sense of security; feeling safe is fundamental to the bottom's ability to abandon himself or herself to the incomparable experience that is sexual rapture.

Erotic restraint is not solely for the bottom's satisfaction, however; the provision of pleasure is a great aphrodisiac—this, combined with the effects of erotic restraint's power shift, empowers the top with a potent sexual force. The responsibility demanded of the top, who agrees to restrain the bottom, is sustained by a surge of adrenaline; it heightens the top's concentration and sense of well-being—which is perhaps also fueled by the awareness that an appeased bottom will be all the more ready and willing to show the full extent of their gratitude when finally set free!

INNER RHYTHM: EROTIC HEARING RESTRAINT

It is difficult if not impossible to achieve complete auditory isolation, so the fruits of temporary hearing deprivation are subtler than those associated with movement and visual restraint. If you are a bottom and your hearing is restrained, you will find that every other sensation will become magnified because of this inward focus, the impact of every stroke that your lover makes heightened. You will hear the sound of your own breathing and your heart beating to the rhythm of the ritual. Such interior sounds augment the meditative effects of ecstasy.

The top's hands will suffice for intermittent hearing restraint, although no doubt the top would rather be busy with his or her hands elsewhere! Earplugs make this possible; those made of soft, pliable balls of beeswax are more effective and comfortable than those of foam or rubber.

Another approach is to dominate the bottom's sense of hearing through sound, with a carefully chosen repertoire of music and headphones. Studies have shown that music we enjoy promotes the production of dopamine—the "feel-good" hormone and neurotransmitter. While the meditative effects of hearing restraint may be slightly reduced with music, it will still serve to accent the effects of a session. Ideally, the top should be able to hear the music, too, but he or she should not wear headphones—the top must hear his or her restrained lover to stay in tune with the bottom.

Certain genres of music are more conducive to sexual transcendence than others. Songs with words, especially if the restrained bottom knows them well, are guaranteed to become a distraction and could inhibit the bottom from concentrating on pleasure alone. Ambient, jazz, and classical music are more likely to facilitate a lover's ability to concentrate on the sensations that are being offered. No matter your musical preference, once the headphones are comfortably in place, confirm that the volume is set just right.

ANTICIPATION: EROTIC SIGHT RESTRAINT

Consider the often extraordinary perceptive capacities of the blind. In order for the brains of the visually impaired to decipher sensory information and compensate for their missing sense, their remaining senses function on acute levels. The unsighted are renowned for being able to hear seemingly imperceptible sounds and distinguish subtle tastes and smells. Their sense of touch is so highly developed that it permits them to read Braille, and even write, thanks to today's technology.

Erotic sight restraint can be practiced to ecstatic effect during any phase of the Sexual Ceremony and in combination with any other form of stimulation. Temporarily depriving the bottom of the ability to see can provoke a powerful psychosensorial charge and bring a rousing element of surprise to the dynamics of the Paradise Found Sexual Ceremony, as the brain does not differentiate between the anticipated sensation and a provided sensation. Concocting the session so that the bottom does not see the tools or have a notion of the sensations that might be offered will prevent the bottom's brain from preparing the body for the receipt of these sensations in advance, heightening the impact of every sensation that the top has in store for the blindfolded bottom.

Slip into Darkness: A Self-Initiation
Erotic sight restraint can be administered most effectively with a blindfold (see plate X, page 170). If you do not wish to invest in a manufactured blindfold, a long piece of silk or a satin scarf will work equally well. Novices to sight restraint may wish to blindfold themselves before giving away or taking the reins of blindfolded pleasure, in order to get an idea of its potential. Dedicate twenty-five to thirty minutes to this exercise to attain insight into its powerful effects.

Lie down or sit in a comfortable position, then tie, buckle, snap, or strap the blindfold snugly into place. Because even the slightest infiltration of light will diminish the impact of the deprivation, the blindfold should impose complete darkness. The eyes are extremely delicate organs, so do not use force in tightening the blindfold. Rest the wrappings against the orbital bone, never against the eyeballs themselves.

Once you are comfortable, allow yourself to ease into the total darkness the blindfold imposes. One of the first things you will notice is that your mind is like a monkey; your thoughts will jump randomly from one place to another. However, in a matter of minutes you will slip into the calm and focused state inherent to the emission of the alpha brain-wave frequency. Practice this self-initiation in silence, without music, to highlight the meditative effects.

Become aware of the sounds around you. They will penetrate what you may have formerly perceived as silence. Focus your attention inward, leave the world behind, and caress yourself. During this sensual meditation, discover the fine, sensitive skin of your lips, your neck, your breasts or chest. Entice your nipples to rise to the occasion before continuing your gradual descent to the sacred source of the sexual vibration.

If you are a man and spending the evening on your own, peak repeatedly. When you finally allow yourself to lose control, the effects of the blindfold will be revealed. If you plan to spend the evening in good company, consider this a preliminary to the shared pleasures that lie ahead, riding the crest of the orgasmic waves and refraining from ejaculating.

If you are a woman, follow the same directions, but accept your orgasm at the end of the experiment, whether you are expecting sweet company or not. It will provide for a blissful release of sexual tension and prepare you for the shared pleasures that lie ahead.

Turn Your Lover On—and Up: A Blindfold Session
The blindfold will augment the perceptual capacity of all of the unrestrained senses, not only the sense of touch, so be prepared to stroke all your partner's senses with erotic intent. Alongside a feather tickler, a horsehair whip or a soft flogger, a pair of latex gloves, a vibrator, and a bottle of lubrication, for example, include the bottom's favorite perfume or essential oil, a piece of chocolate, or some slices of juicy fruit—anything that you know will turn your

lover on—and up—can be used to tantalize his or her senses.

Invite the bottom to lie, sit, or go onto all fours; his or her position will depend on the pleasures that the top intends to provide. Once your lover is comfortable, put the blindfold in place. Confirm that it is not causing discomfort and that the bottom is in total darkness. If the bottom is also to be subject to movement restraint, the blindfold should be put on *after* he or she has been bound.

From this moment on, you must be prepared to remain in close contact with the bottom at all times. Before proceeding, grant the bottom a few moments of silence. This will permit you both to focus your thoughts, before the session commences. It will also allow the bottom to adjust to the effects of the power shift.

Adopt a calm, quiet tone of voice. If music is being played, turn down its volume. Visual restraint augments our perception of sound. As soon as the bottom has slipped into the calm, relaxed mindset, he or she will be ready to focus on pleasure. Before long the bottom will be writhing in anticipation, quivering to your every touch and begging for more. You might whisper your sweetest intentions into the bottom's ears, then, rather than meeting their ecstatic expectations immediately, take the long way around—building sweet anticipation mounts sexual tension even higher!

As the ceremony gradually progresses, the psychophysiological effects of sight deprivation will begin to manifest. The impact of every touch, tickle, lick, scratch, kiss, squeeze, spank, and loving caress will be reinforced by every sexy sound, taste, and scent that you as the top conjure up. The ritual's harmonious progression will transform the bottom into a highly sensitized, receptive, and even downright submissive playmate. The more creative freedom you have and, of course, the more sexually skilled and in tune with your lover's needs you are, the more relaxed and receptive the bottom will become, and the more fun and exciting the session will be for both of you.

Avoid administering too many different kinds of sensations during the same session. The blindfolded bottom's heightened state of arousal and receptivity is a direct reflection of his or her physical and emotional hypersensitivity, so to avoid creating sensory confusion, it is important that you channel acute mental and physical presence. Before long, neither you nor the bottom will be able to resist the need to soothe your mutual, aching desire.

If your bottom is male, only if the timing is right should he be allowed to ejaculate. Otherwise, you should redirect his attention, either by focusing on another area of his body or by privileging another sense. For example, you may opt to serve him something delicious—say a spoonful of his favorite ice cream. It will not only smell and taste more heavenly but also feel colder than ever before. Erotic sight restraint enhances thermoception, so tease your bottom's warm lips, plump with arousal, with the back of the cold spoon before asking him or her to open wide for an explosion of flavor!

If you are playing on a hot summer's day, put a bowl of ice cubes at hand's reach. On a cold winter's night, hot wax play may be equally appreciated. Combining temperature play with the effects of the blindfold makes for all the more sizzling a session!

If the blindfold is removed midsession, be prepared to enjoy gathering the fruits of the bottom's generosity; your lover will be in an ecstatic state, eager to return and share the heightened pleasure. Caress, touch, tease, and please each other until neither of you can take any more! If the blindfold is removed toward the end of the Sexual Ceremony, join the restrained bottom to climb the summits of pleasure together, and relish the earth-trembling consequences. As the session ends, warn the bottom before removing the blindfold—otherwise the unexpected flash of light may cause him or her to crash rather than sweetly glide from Paradise back to reality!

INTIMATE BONDS: EROTIC MOVEMENT RESTRAINT

Bondage is one of the most common sexual fantasies for women and men alike. Those who choose to explore the powers of erotic movement restraint consider it to be liberating, creative, and empowering. Its capacity to reinforce the bonds of intimacy by revealing, pushing, and permitting lovers to hurdle sexual boundaries is renowned.

There are many ways to restrain the consenting lover's movement, but this section focuses on verbal bondage, cuffs, and cords. Being that the art of rope bondage demands skill as well as diligent practice in order to reach its ecstatic ends, a separate section of this chapter is dedicated to those techniques.

No matter how it is achieved, bondage can be practiced in combination with other forms of stimulation. For example, some bondage aficionados enjoy being penetrated while bound. Others prefer the pleasures of bondage to penetration itself. Some revel in being deprived of their sense of movement in combination with other forms of erotic restraint, while for others this prompts sensory overload. Those who enjoy erotic tickling or flagellation may like to be bound for the occasion. From a purely practical point of view, this last scenario avoids the risk that the bottom may involuntarily hurt himself or herself or the top with an unexpected gesture of excitement. Others may find that high-impact extra-genital stimulation, like flagellation, becomes too intense if administered while they are physically restrained. Experience alone can reveal what works best, whether we are binding or bound. No matter how much experience partners may have or how hard they like to play, lovers should always progress gradually toward the more challenging forms of restraint.

Novices especially should refrain from combining movement restraint with other forms of sensory deprivation until they have acquired some practice in bondage skills and understood its myriad effects. Novices should engage in "soft" bondage until they acquire more experience. "Hard" bondage, as its name implies, is more rigorous and demanding. Soft bondage entails natural and therefore more comfortable positions, and in soft bondage scenes, the bottom may even be able to set himself or herself free with only a little effort. Some bondage aficionados consider such Houdini-esque attempts to escape an integral part of bondage fun. Hard bondage makes such attempts next to impossible. But bondage does not have to be hard to incite transcendental results. In fact, being bound at length in comfortable positions can provoke ecstatic results—as long as the top is prepared to take the bottom to Paradise!

Whether bondage is the leitmotif or an ecstatic highlight of the Sexual Ceremony, the top and the bottom are equally responsible for the final outcome of the session. It is crucial that both partners come into the temple relaxed, well rested, and ready to transcend. Both should have eaten a light meal, no less than two hours before. Interrupting the digestive cycle is dangerous, and it should be avoided at all costs. Light, fresh, high-energy foods and plenty of water will energize the body; fatty foods and carbohydrates require more energy to be digested and can leave one feeling sluggish. Neither the top nor bottom should practice any movement restraint when not feeling perfectly physically and emotionally well.

Even partners who know each other well ought to review the boundaries of a bondage session before the Sexual Ceremony starts. The more skills and experience that lovers acquire, the more likely they are to enjoy "programming" the session's progression, particularly when assuming the role of top. As with erotic sight restraint, once the bottom's bonds are in place, the top is obliged to stay in near-constant physical contact. This is as crucial to the bottom's capacity to surrender as it is to his or her safety. Remember that sensory deprivation incites a certain degree of physical and emotional vulnerability, so only if the bottom feels safe and secure in submitting to his or her partner will the final outcome of the session be positively thrilling.

Bondage has been described as "motion in stillness." As passive as the bottom may appear to be to the eyes of the inexperienced, bondage demands both outer and inner strength; the more intense the restraint, the more endurance, flexibility, and determination is required. These virtues will become all the more relevant in the more physically demanding variations of rope bondage. When the bottom consents to more extreme degrees of movement restraint, he or she should do a minimum of stretching to warm up muscles. This will enhance circulation and reduce the likelihood of cramping, sprains, and strains, as well as increasing the bottom's overall resistance to greater degrees of restraint and constriction. The more effectively the restraint is imposed, the longer the bottom may remain bound, and the faster sexual tension will mount.

BEFORE THE REVEL, REMEMBER . . .

Tops and bottoms must attempt not only a physical but also an emotional symbiosis throughout the ceremony. What this means is that while it is the responsibility of the top to provide for his or her bound partner, it is the bottom's vital duty to check in on himself or herself as well, no matter how high each is flying. The bottom must not hold the top entirely responsible for his or her physical, emotional, and spiritual well-being. Even a bottom who usually enjoys bondage may feel neither physically nor emotionally open enough to revel in its powers.

The longer a bottom is restrained, the more he or she will struggle. An instinctive response to movement restraint, it serves to minimize discomfort and is an integral part of the fun and pleasure. It makes the heart beat faster, prompting the blood to flow more readily toward the surface of the skin, heightening the bottom's overall sensitivity. It also further increases endorphin production. But the more intensely the ceremony evolves, the more attentive the top must be to ensure a harmonious outcome.

The top must keep in mind that once a consenting lover has been bound, his or her overall perceptions, and, therefore, sensitivity will be radically enhanced. The top must exercise self-control—the more gradually the top builds the shared sexual tension, the more both partners will be charged—body, mind, and spirit—with the sexual vibration.

When bondage is the leitmotif of the sexual ceremony, the partner that bottomed can, if so inclined, provide his or her top with similar pleasures during the next phase of the ceremony—reversing roles, in essence. (Do allow the bottom to enjoy coming down from the peaks of the endorphin high after he or she has been set free and before the switch.) But consider that the longer and more all encompassing the session is, the more consolidated the roles of top and bottom are likely to become. Inverting the dynamics of the power shift may therefore not be convenient or feel natural for either partner. But keep the option open—lovers should follow their instincts, and let their sense of sexual freedom and creativity soar!

OBEY!: EROTIC VERBAL RESTRAINT

When the bottom is simultaneously being caressed, licked, tickled, cropped, or spanked to delight, he or she is likely to have a hard time obeying the top's orders . . . and this is where the fun begins! The practice of verbal bondage is the safest form of erotic restraint; it simply entails telling an aroused lover not to move. If a partner is aroused and fully immersed in the sexual dimension, and at the right time and in the right context they are told, "Do not move, not even an inch," it will make a strong psychophysiological impact.

Prior to making an investment in any bondage gear, bondage

novices can test each other's receptivity to movement restraint with this simple technique. (It also travels well!) Lovers who enjoy its effects are very likely to succumb to the powers and potential that the instruments of erotic movement restraint can provide. But novices who do not respond well to verbal bondage should not feel or be obliged to engage in this or any other technique of movement restraint.

"BOUND" TO BE SATISFIED: BONDAGE CUFFS

Bondage cuffs and their related accessories are both easy to obtain and to employ. To get started, invest in a basic bondage cuff set composed of two ankle cuffs, two wrists cuffs, and four snap-hooks or S-hooks. I recommend that you choose high-quality cuffs in soft, padded leather; while they may be more costly, they are wildly more comfortable than those made of stiff belt leather. High-quality cuffs will not scratch or chafe the fine skin of the wrists and ankles, and they do a better job of reducing the risk of strains or sprains. The more comfortable the cuffs, the longer your bondage sessions can last, and the more satisfying the end results are bound to be—no pun intended!

Any bondage cuff made of metal may cause injury, should it be subject to tension or strain during the course of a bondage session. Because undue discomfort may distract the bottom from concentrating on his or her pleasure, avoid using real handcuffs unless they are necessary to reinforce the psychological impact of certain kinds of role-play. If you and your lover like the idea of locking someone up tight, or being locked up, soft, padded leather cuffs will serve the purpose.

Do not, however, underestimate the psychological impact that locks and keys have. They are potent symbols of sexual possession, and while some lovers appreciate their capacity to reinforce the role of top and bottom, others will feel claustrophobic at the mere idea of being locked in. Should you and your partner choose to use restraints with padlocks, the top must keep the keys at hand's reach or, better yet, on a chain around his or her neck. For the bottom, the sight of the keys dangling from the chain will act as a constant reminder that his or her only duty is to surrender to the pleasure that the top has in store.

Ideally, the same key should open all of the locks, but in the case that it does not, each lock and its relative key should be color-coded. A top fumbling with his or her keys will not instill a sense security in a bound bottom who has asked to be set free. Without losing his or her sense (or appearance) of being calm and in control, the top will want to respond immediately to avoid anxiety or resistance in the bottom.

THE SHIFT OF POWER: A BONDAGE SESSION WITH CUFFS

Movement restraint can be used during any phase of the Sexual Ceremony's evolution. If you are the top, begin the session by restraining the bottom's hands at the front of his or her body, a position that permits the bottom to access his or her own genitals. If hands are bound at the back, this will be impossible, and the shift of power into your hands will be more complete. Once the wrists or ankles cuffs are in place, ensure that they are tight enough to prevent the bottom's hands or feet from slipping out of them but not so tight that they chafe the skin or, worse, compromise blood circulation.

After having verified the bottom's comfort, invite the bottom to lie, kneel, or sit down before restraining his or her ankles. (The ankles must never be bound directly to each other if the bottom is in an upright position, unless the upper body is fully supported or the bottom is able to brace firmly against a stable object like a chair or a table. Failure to respect this rule can put your bottom in danger of toppling over.)

If the bottom is a woman, penetration will be next to impossible if her ankles are bound and she is positioned facing her top. A skilled top will use this inaccessibility to the bottom's benefit and take advantage of the power of anticipation to enhance the final impact of pleasure. But before long, you both are likely to be possessed with raging desire, and you may decide to either roll the bottom onto the front of her body, which will grant entry to her secret garden of delight, or change her position altogether by restraining, for example, the bottom's wrists to her ankles. (The ability to change a bottom's position with ease and in a matter of seconds is one great advantage of bondage cuffs and their attached snap hooks.) This position is also known as "the crab"; it grants easy access to the sacred source of the sexual vibration, whether the bottom is a man or a woman, facing the top or not.

Note that, like any position that forces the bottom to fully expose his or her genitals and anal area, the crab can be a source of humiliation. While ritualized humiliation may be a source of arousal for some, not everyone appreciates its effects.

FULL CONTROL: BONDAGE POSITIONS

Partners who enjoy the effects of basic cuff-to-cuff restraint may eventually wish to expand their repertoire by investing in a few extra accessories. Bondage straps, which can be purchased through any BDSM supplier, will make for some exciting alternatives to basic cuff-to-cuff restraint. They can be used to bind the bottom spread-eagled either face-up or face-down on the bed (see plate IX, page 169) or to impose, for example, what is commonly known as "the hog-tie" (see plate X, page 170). Due to its theatrical appeal, this bondage position is commonly represented in BDSM and alternative erotic magazines and literature, as well as by the film industry. The hog-tie is decidedly dynamic, demanding in the bottom a certain degree of strength and flexibility, if not a good dose of highly aroused determination in order to rest in its embrace even for short periods. Because the hog-tie's psychophysiological impact is acute, lovers should gradually work their way up to its practice. The spread-eagle position is, on the other hand, relatively comfortable and excellent for lengthy restraint. It can also be performed in an upright position.

Prepare for what I call "the standing eagle" by mounting two sturdy eye-screws or swivel hooks on the upper and lower left- and right-hand sides of a wooden door frame, wall, or other sturdy support. Make certain the hardware and the support are solid enough to bear the weight and stress of the bottom's struggles. Swivel hooks provide the advantage of "giving" and moving with the bottom's motions, thereby reducing the risk of injuries.

The bottom's position will be determined by the pleasures that the top has planned. If the bottom is bound facing the door or wall, you, as the top, will have access to the back and buttocks, which is a prime opportunity to provide a wide range of extra-genital pleasures—from erotic tickling to flagellation—as well as genital and anal stimulation. If the bottom is bound facing you, the genitals, breasts, nipples, and mouth are the principal points of focus, as the joys of erotic flagellation can only be provided safely to certain areas of the body, as described in the chapter "*X* Marks the Sweet Spot: Erotic Flagellation."

After the wrist cuffs have been secured to the eye-hooks, you may proceed, if you wish, to hook the bottom's ankles either together or apart (if eye-hooks have also been installed at ankle level). If you desire to take more control of the bottom's movements, a spreader bar can be used to force the bottom's feet apart, about shoulders' width. This device is usually attached to the ankles by means of cuffs, and it significantly reinforces the dynamics of the standing spread-eagle restraint, as well as the those of the rest of the session, as it grants the top full control over the now very accessible genitals! Note that when you decide to release or change the bottom's standing position, his or her ankles must be released first, so the bottom's balance is not compromised.

DANGEROUS MOVES

At the turn of the twenty-first century, advertising experts began to use decontextualized bondage imagery to promote a wide variety of commodities, from alcoholic beverages to handbags, pasta to bathroom tiles. Americans may remember a campaign that came out in September 2008 representing actress Jessica Alba being physically and restrained and gagged by bondage tape, and to promote a very good cause—encouraging young people to vote!

But another advertising campaign was launched for a less politically correct motive—to promote a world-famous cocktail mixer. The advertisement unwittingly also promoted some glaringly dangerous bondage mistakes, which I will use to highlight four fundamental bondage-safety guidelines.

A very young model wearing a string bikini is seated in a chair in front of a low glass table at the edge of a pool. Her wrists are bound to the armrests of the chair, one wrist with a necktie, the other with a leather belt. Her eyelids, half-closed seductively, are heavy with aquamarine eye shadow. Her red lips are parted with desire. But if this young bottom found herself in this position during a real bondage session, not on a photo set, she would have several very good reasons to feel insecure and even frightened, and her expression would reflect anything *but* sexual readiness.

The first reason is that there is not even a shadow to be seen of the person who bound her. *Safety guideline #1*: Leaving a bound partner alone can put them in real danger—at the very least incite cathartic and anything but erotic reactions. Tops, you must honor your bottoms by keeping them safe with your attentive presence.

The second danger represented in the image is the bound model's proximity to the glass table and the deceptively placid waters of the pool. *Safety guideline #2*: The temple of erotic loving, whether it is erected indoors or out, must be arranged to guarantee the safety and well-being of both partners. On a scale of one to ten, the risk involved in this scenario is eleven, as a bound lover is guaranteed to struggle. If this damsel struggled, she could fall, face forward, into the glass table, or sideways into the swimming pool.

The third faux pas represented by the image is the association of movement restraint with alcohol. *Safety guideline #3*: Bondage combined with alcoholic beverages, or any other mind-altering substance, can make for a very dangerous cocktail. Alcohol inhibits one's sense of judgment, as well as one's overall perception of pleasure, as it masks the exhilarating effects of endorphin elation.

The fourth risk represented by the image is one commonly depicted by media, literature, and film. While I cannot deny the aesthetic and symbolic appeal of using men's silk ties and leather belts, these are inappropriate bondage tools. Belts are not perforated in the correct place for wrist or ankle restraint, so for bondage they are neither comfortable nor effective. A man's necktie can be used as a blindfold, but silky materials make slippery knots that can tighten under strain. As the bottom struggles, the tighter these silky knots will become, and the more dangerously difficult they are to untie. In the case of an emergency, the top will be obliged to cut this strip of haberdashery in two. *Safety guideline #4*: Always use bondage gear designed specifically for the purpose of safe and pleasurable erotic restraint. It will enhance the overall quality and safety of your bondage sessions.

This kind of advertising imagery utilizes shock value, the exploitation of which, in this case, perpetuates and glamorizes sexual ignorance. Perhaps one day information beneficial to sexual health and well-being will suffuse advertising's bondage imagery. Ad execs will

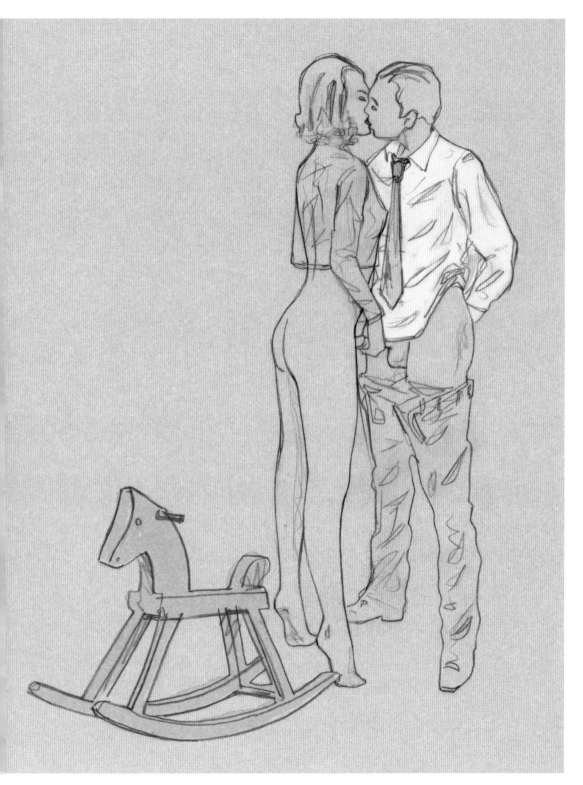

PLATE XVII THE CEREMONY COMMENCES

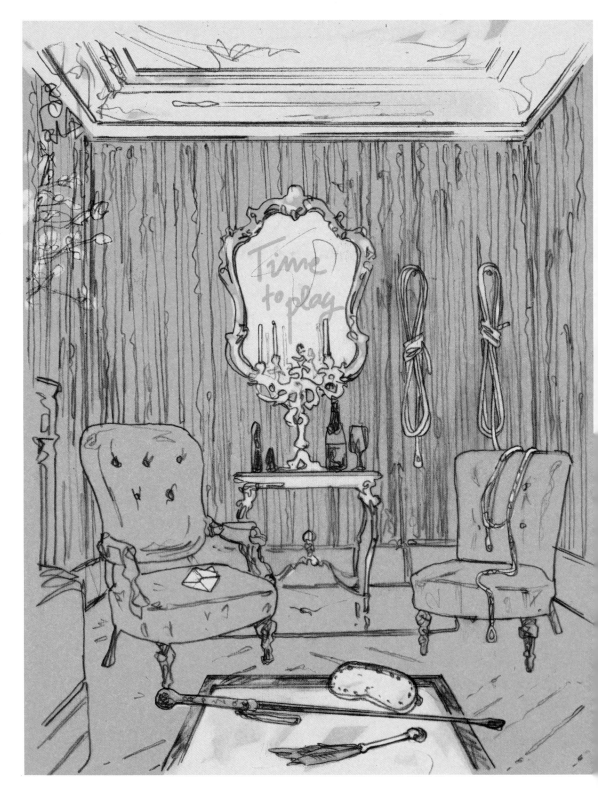

PLATE XVIII THE TEMPLE

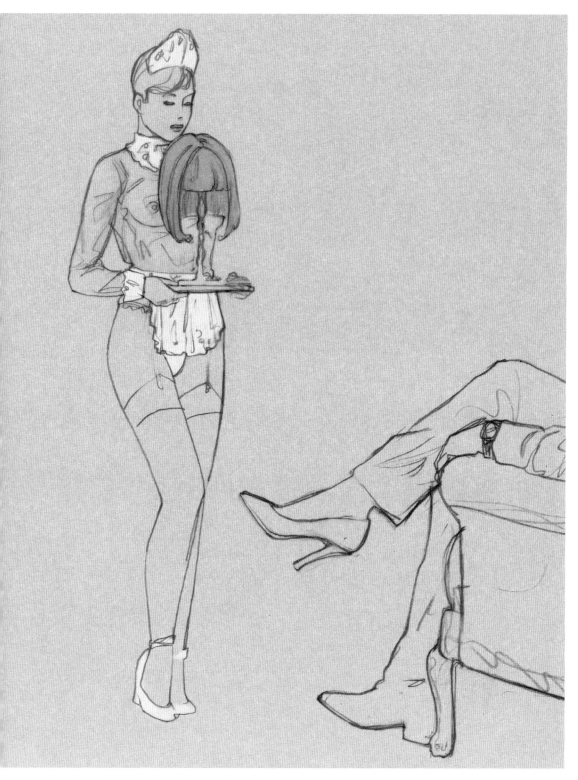

PLATE XIX CEREMONY WITH ROLE-PLAY

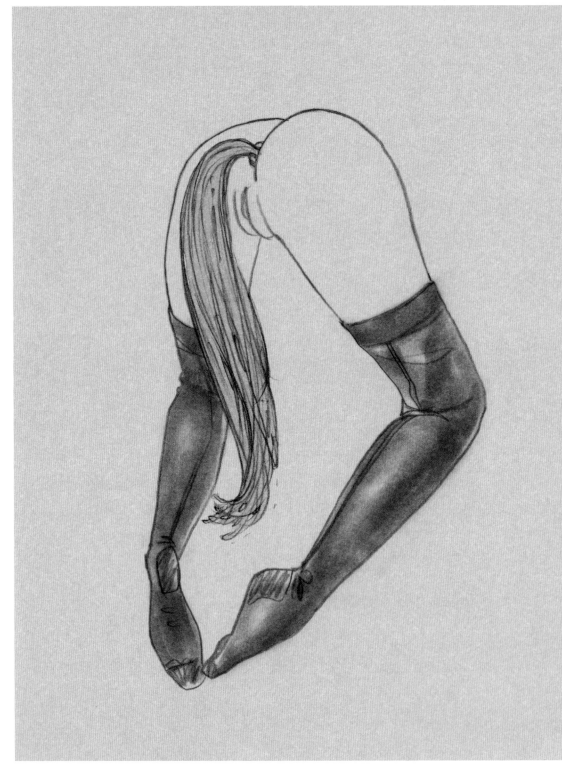

PLATE XX PONY PLAY WITH HORSETAIL WHIP AS ANAL TOOL

then discover that the promise of real pleasure can be an even more effective marketing tool.

THE ULTIMATE BOND: SENSUAL ROPE BONDAGE

Adventurous lovers who enjoy testing and pushing their sexual limits consider sensual rope bondage the ultimate in erotic restraint. Whether wielding or yielding to the powers of the cords, aficionados of rope bondage laud its capacity to reinforce the sexual bond.

Cords permit for a wider range and degree of restraint than bondage cuffs. Sensual rope bondage, when masterfully executed, imbues a consenting bottom with sexuality, vulnerability, and strength. This, along with the technique's capacity to make endorphins surge, builds unexpected levels of sexual tension that lead to radically heightened levels of arousal.

In ancient Japan, the art of sensual rope bondage was traditionally known as *kinbaku*, meaning "tight binding." Practitioners of kinbaku considered the tying of knots on the human body to be unacceptable, even vulgar. Consequentially, in its purest, most unadulterated form, the technique calls for very few knots to attain its highly aesthetic and sensual purpose. Today, the Japanese style of bondage is more commonly known as *shibari*, from the verb "to tie." Shibari combines the techniques of binding and tying, and its artistry serves the Japanese on an everyday basis, not just for erotic purposes—from tying a lowly package to ornamental food preparation to the arrangement of beautiful kimonos. Masters of kinbaku and shibari consider sharing the beauty of their bindings part of the pleasure these arts provides; thus, sensual rope bondage is practiced not only privately but also publicly, as a form of adult entertainment.

In the West the practice of sensual rope bondage, public or private, is largely confined to the BDSM community. Though easy Internet access to directions and videos makes the uninitiated think they might practice rope bondage with impunity, there are real risks involved. In order to tap into the erotic potential of cords, lovers must refine their bondage skills through practice. Lovers who are unable to invest the time and energy to learn basic techniques should restrict themselves to the use of bondage cuffs and the related accessories explored in the previous section.

THE "NO" ZONES

Before we take the kinks out of the cords, it is important to highlight the "no" zones of the body for safe rope bondage (see plate IX, page 169): the front of the neck, the armpits, the groin, the inner crook of elbows and knees, and the pulse points of ankles and wrists.

While the back of the neck can support a certain degree of pressure, the front of the neck is the number one "no" zone. Do not ever wrap cords around a lover's neck or apply any pressure at all to the front of this delicate region of the body. Pressure on the front of the neck will compromise the breathing; it takes only a few minutes of pressure to cause injury or even death.

Other "no" zones are the armpits and the groin; both areas house major blood vessels and delicate glands and should, therefore, never be subject to pressure. Neither should the fine-skinned inner crook of the elbow or knee be compressed; their delicate blood vessels and nerves lie very close to the surface of the skin.

The delicate articulations of the wrists and the ankles, where veins also lie so close to the surface that they are visible, should never be bound with rope directly on their pulse points. Wrap slightly *above* or *below* the pulse point. Whenever the position of the bottom permits, when binding wrists, press them together, pulse point to pulse point, to further reduce the risk of injury.

When the wrists or ankles are bound at length, periodically the top should ask the bottom to wriggle his or her fingers and/or toes from time to time, in order to verify that their circulation is not being compromised. (This will also remind the bottom to check in on himself or herself, even when flying high.)

But while the "no" zones should never be compressed or put under strain, they are highly erogenous and will grow all the more receptive to being sweetly teased and tantalized, once the bottom is bound.

THE DANCE OF THE CORDS

Sophisticated knots are fun to master and pleasing to the eye, but they aren't essential to basic sensual rope bondage. Knots that are easy to release and that do not tighten over the bottom's flesh when they are put under strain are, on the other hand, fundamental to safe, sensual practice.

Harmonious binding of any permitted body part is also essential to bondage safety. A haphazard crossing of ropes will not only create discomfort but also bruise and chafe the skin, dangerously inhibit circulation, injure the articulations at wrists and ankles, and even cause permanent damage to nerve endings. The dance of the cords should result in harmonious, well-balanced bindings that are tight enough so the bound partner cannot get free but loose enough to permit the top to slide two fingers between the cords and the bottom's skin. Integrating this test into the ceremony after every binding that you finish should become automatic. If a bottom ever feels that a restraint is too tight or not quite right, he or she needs to inform the top immediately so that it can be adjusted. While most bondage aficionados consider the temporary marks that snug ropes leave on the skin as one of the technique's inherent pleasures, marks caused by rope burn may be considered less endearing—and are also more enduring. Such "souvenirs" from Paradise can be avoided if the top places his or her fingers between the moving cord and the bottom's skin.

Masters of sensual rope bondage channel the forces of balance and beauty throughout every phase of a bondage session. Strive to do the same—and your bondage efforts will result in mutual satisfaction in no time. Aesthetics are to be considered an integral aspect of the pleasures that bondage provides for both partners. Ideally, mirrors should be strategically placed in the ritual space to permit both the top and the bottom to view their ceremonial endeavors.

The Slip and Slither of the Cords
Shopping for ropes can be an inspirational preliminary to the Sexual Ceremony. Every bondage aficionado has a rope of preference, and you will discover through practice the virtues of each one. The distinct sensations that a cord provides as it slips and slithers across a bottom's skin is an important part of the pleasures of bondage. The material that bondage cords are made of, as well as the speed at which they move as the restraint is being executed, will imbue each session with unique sensations. Those who have acquired some degree of sensual bondage skills may wish to invest in a proper set of precut and conditioned bondage cords, as well as a few lessons with a master.

Nylon ropes are good for novice efforts, as they are easy to come by and less expensive than quality cotton, linen, or hemp ropes. Cords made from these organic materials are also far more pleasant for the top to maneuver than synthetic ones, and the bottom will appreciate their natural, sensual touch. Those made of silk and its synthetic imitations are even more sensual in feel as they slither and glide across the bottom's skin—unfortunately, they have the disadvantage of making slippery knots and bindings that are likely to slide and cross each other and even come undone.

Lovers of sensual rope bondage often prefer rope made from hemp for its organic aesthetic appeal and the sensual, earthy scent it unleashes. When under strain, hemp rope makes a distinct "creaking" sound that has a sensuous impact. And, very important, the knots in hemp ropes are easy to release, even when tight. Hemp will soften with washing and can be treated with beeswax or rope conditioners that will increase the life span of the ropes.

Some bondage lovers prefer twisted rather than braided cords, as they leave more distinct marks on the skin. These ceremonial mementos normally vanish an hour or so after the cords have been removed. However, cords that are woven or braided make for a better investment, because they won't unravel and are generally more resistant to washing.

No matter the material, make sure whatever rope you buy does not have a wire core. When this kind of rope becomes worn, its wire may be exposed, which could injure either partner. In addition, bondage cords must be kept clean. Hygiene is as relevant to these tools as to any other erotic instrument, and it becomes all the more relevant should you use the same cords with different partners. When cords are used repeatedly, they eventually show signs of wear and tear; worn, frayed cords risk snapping in two if they are employed to support even the slightest degree of weight or pressure. Cords that are not in good condition should thus be considered dangerous and replaced, not only for safety but also for aesthetic reasons.

Compress, Hug, and Caress: A Basic Rope Bondage Kit
A basic rope bondage kit comprises approximately 130 feet (40 meters) of cord. Quality rope is not cheap, so don't invest in large quantities until you are certain that you and your partner will make good use of it. There is always time to make a trip back to the local hardware store, nautical shop, or erotic supplier as you refine your skill in creating more intricate, sophisticated, and effective movement-restricting bonds.

The rope you choose should be $\frac{5}{16}$ inches (8 millimeters) in diameter. It will make for flat, aesthetically pleasing, and easily released knots—if they are tied properly in the first place! Bondage masters may use a wider variety of diameters, depending on the kinds of bondage to be done, but ¼-inch (6-millimeter) rope is considered to be the minimum diameter required for safe sensual rope bondage. Thinner rope may cut into the bottom's skin when put under even a slight degree of strain. It also makes for small, hard-to-release knots that are not nearly as aesthetically pleasing as those tied in slightly thicker rope.

Divide your rope into sections of varying lengths. Rope approximately 8 feet long (2.5 meters) is ideal for binding the hands together. Rope approximately 12 feet in length (3.5 meters) is perfect for binding the ankles together as well as for binding the wrists directly to the ankles. Two sections of approximately 26 feet (8 meters) and 40 feet (12 meters) in length can be used for making chest harnesses and other delightful variations on shibari that not only restrain and restrict the bottom's sense of movement but compress, hug, and caress large areas of the body as well.

Once you have cut the rope, don't put the scissors away. You still need to seal the ends of the rope in order to prevent fraying and unraveling. Do not tie knots at the ends of your rope! Their bulk will render your bondage session downright clumsy, if not next to impossible to accomplish.

For nylon rope, wrap the ends of each rope with masking tape, leaving approximately ¼ inch (6 millimeters) of the end exposed to make a clean finish. Heat the blade of a knife over a flame then rub the hot blade over the ends of the rope. Once is has cooled, remove and discard the tape. Heating the ends of nylon rope can make their edges rough; fine sandpaper can be used to soften any sharp, scratchy edges. Another solution is to use masking or electrical tape alone to prevent the rope from unraveling.

The ends of rope made from natural materials like hemp, linen, or cotton are traditionally "whipped," or bound and stitched with twine, to prevent them from fraying, but they, too, can just be wrapped with masking tape. However, this makes for a less visually pleasing bondage cord, no matter the material in question. Consider binding or even stitching the ends of the rope with colored thread to obtain a more visually pleasing result—aesthetics should never be forgotten. I cap my own cords with smooth metal tips, which prevent fraying and add a slight weight to the working ends that facilitates the knotting and binding process. They also bejewel my bondage cords, adding a distinct aesthetic benefit to their erotic function. Take a trip to the hardware store—where unexpected bondage solutions await your sexually creative mind!

Everyone knows that a rope has two ends, but in order to benefit from the initiation in this chapter, you must understand the language of the bondage cords a bit more extensively. The length of the cord that lies between the ends is called the *standing line*. This section is usually involved in the binding process but not the knotting. The *main line* marks the beginning of the knot, which terminates with the *working end* of the cord. The main line is usually kept taut until the knot is tied with the working end. A *loop* is created when a cord is folded back and crosses over itself. A *hitch* is a knot that ties a cord to something else, like a hook. Because a hitch tightens under strain, it should not be used directly on the bindings that constrict your happy lover.

Once the ends of the ropes are prepped, find the center of each rope and mark it with a colored thread, a waterproof pen, or a piece of tape. This will permit the top to find the middle of the bondage cord instantly, contributing to the control and fluidity of every gesture made when working with doubled cords. Many of the restraints to be explored are executed with doubled cords; this permits for faster binds and lends more support to the bound limbs and also imbues the binds with a very distinct, pleasing aesthetic.

Plan ahead and color-code these center marks to indicate cord length; for example, use black to indicate 26 feet (8 meters), red for 12 feet (3.5 meters), and so forth. To bundle and store your bondage cords, fold each length in half and, holding the center loop in one hand, repeatedly wrap around the elbow and the palm until the entire length of the cord is in an orderly ring. Then loop, tie, or twist the ends of the cord around the ring to prevent it from unraveling. Now it is ready for titillating action!

Good organization is crucial to every phase of sensual rope bondage. Being organized means the top isn't undoing kinks and knots instead of dedicating attention to pleasure; it supports the meditative trance-state that the harmonious dance of the cords will evoke in both partners. Some bottoms enjoy taking care of the ropes before the session starts; in fact, their tops can insist that the bottom does so! The partner who is responsible for this phase of the ceremony should make sure that the cords are clean, note wear and tear, and replace any defective cords with a new one.

Once the cords are doubled and neatly bundled, they should be set out in an orderly fashion next to the instruments that will be used to coax the bottom through the gates of Paradise. The top must also remember to keep a pair of blunt-nosed medical shears within arm's reach to quickly release a bound bottom in case he or she is in any danger.

Being Present at the Gates of Paradise
The safety guidelines that were set forth in the previous section on bondage cuffs should be followed in combination with those below that pertain specifically to sensual rope bondage.

The heightened states of sexual arousal that are intrinsic to the arts of rope bondage depend on factors that go beyond the ability of the top to orchestrate the dance of the cords. For example, the top must *stay in physical contact with the bottom at all times.*

The top's presence, like his or her touch, instills a sense of security that helps trigger sexual abandon in the bottom. Coaxing the bottom toward the gates of Paradise with the hands and fingers also permits the top to make certain that the constricted areas of the bottom's body are staying warm. Should any part of a bottom's body go cold, it is a sign that his or her circulation is compromised.

Should the bottom experience numbness or a tingling sensation, the ropes must be removed at once. Do not wait until the bottom is unable to feel or move the body part in question; once the bottom is freed from the cords, the top should then massage the affected areas and help the bottom flex the numbed body part to encourage the return of circulation.

The most extreme variations of rope bondage entail total or partial suspension of the body and demand great technical skill in order to be performed safely. It also helps if the bottom is in excellent physical shape and knows his or her physical and emotional limits. The techniques of suspension bondage will not be dealt with in this volume, as they are too complex to be safely taught in a limited context. Anyone who masters the basic restraints taught in this chapter and who wishes to learn the more advanced forms of sensual rope bondage should seek out a master in those arts.

Practice for Pleasure
Due to the dangers inherent to sensual rope bondage, I recommend that novices practice on inanimate objects before inviting a lover to submit to the power of the cords. A medium-size cloth doll or even a teddy bear makes for an ideal bondage-training companion. During the Edo period in Japan (1603–1867), a time of flourishing arts, rope bondage techniques were commonly mastered on straw dummies. Unlike human beings, dolls cannot be put at risk, nor will they feel insecure when trainees fumble with the cord, execute knots that cannot be easily released, or create

restraints that are sloppy, too tight, or downright dangerous. Lovers, take heed: you are bound to make these mistakes until you master the dance of the cords.

When practicing with a medium-size doll, use a cord with the diameter of ¼ inch (6 millimeters). Cut it into lengths of approximately 3 feet, 6 feet, and 10 feet (1, 2, and 3 meters). If you train on yourself, use cords with a ⁵⁄₁₆-inch (8-millimeter) diameter; you will, of course, have to limit your attention to your lower body.

When you feel confident in your skill with the cords, invite a trusted friend or lover to submit to your education. Keep things simple, and progress gradually. Not until you have mastered each restraint that you intend to use, to the point that you feel as if you could almost execute it in your sleep, should you put it to ceremonial use. You and your partner will both benefit from your training; mutual confidence is fundamental to the shared pleasures of sensual rope bondage.

The skilled top is aware that the more restrictive a restraint is, the less likely it is that the bottom will be able to resist in its embrace at length. The top always progresses gradually toward more demanding restraints. Unless the top knows the bottom's physical limits well, the top should not submit the bottom to the more challenging forms of restraint at the beginning, nor impose lengthy periods of immobilization. The bottom should refrain from touching the cords with their hands whenever possible. This will reinforce the positive effects of the power shift, accentuate the fluidity of the top's gestures, and enhance the overall harmony of the session.

Japanese rope bondage is often asymmetrical, but this chapter focuses on basic symmetrical restraints alone—some Western, others in the Japanese style—that provide equal degrees of support, tension, and pressure on both sides of the body. The basic knots explored herein are common to sailors, scouts, rock climbers, and equestrians—not just to lovers of sensual rope bondage.

Snug, Not Tight: Cuffs with the French Bowline

The initiation into sensual rope bondage commences with learning how to create bondage cuffs using a knot known as the French bowline (see plate IX, page 169). All cords are ⁵⁄₁₆ inch (8 millimeters) in diameter. Your 8-foot-long (2.5-meter) cord should be used to bind the wrists; your 12-foot-long (3.5-meter) cord are perfect for binding the ankles.

Start with a single strand of cord and create an overhand loop at one of its ends, making sure to pass the working end of the cord *over*, not under, the main line (the portion of cord that marks the beginning of the knot). The French bowline will otherwise not take shape.

Then, while holding this loop between your fingers in one hand, run the working end of the cord once around the wrist or the ankle and then pull the end through the loop. Repeat this gesture at least three times, but certainly more if desired, in order to create a band of cords. This provides for more comfortable and safer restraints, because should the bottom struggle, the cord's tension will be spread over all the cords; it will also help to avoid chafing. (Remember that struggling and straining is a natural response and part of the endorphin-surging fun of movement restraint!)

In order to terminate each French bowline "cuff," the last time the working end of the cord is looped around the wrist or ankle, its end should be pulled through the loop again. But rather than wrapping it around the limb, run the end directly around the main line (the portion of the cord that marks the very beginning of the knot) and pass it directly back through the loop.

Before tightening the knot, work the cords to take up the slack, making sure that all the loops that go around the limb are of equal length. The final result should be snug, not tight. Slide your forefinger and middle finger between the cords and the bottom's skin to ensure that the delicate pulse points are not under pressure. The French bowline will not slip or tighten, so this danger is unlikely—as long as the knot is tied properly.

Once both the ankles and wrists have been cuffed, all of the bondage cuffs variations explored in the preceding section may be enacted. When the hand-to-hand, ankle-to-ankle, or ankle-to-hand bonds are being implemented, the top must again take care that the French bowlines lie just above or just below the pulse points— never directly on the points. When the wrists and ankles are bound directly to each other, the restraint should be secured with a safety knot for the quick release, if necessary, of the bound bottom.

Please Release Me: The Safety Knot
Fast release is fundamental to safe sensual bondage. There are several variations on the safety knot, but the following is the easiest to remember, as it is as simple as tying as your shoes. The one dif-ference is that the knot is a half bow created with one loop rather than two before the cords are pulled tight. To form a half bow, proceed as if you were tying your shoes. Make the first loop, then the second loop, then begin to tie the bow. As you tighten it, continue pulling the working end of the second loop all the way through and—voilà! Pull taut. This safety knot can be used to secure any binding made directly on the body and can be released in a matter of seconds by pulling on the loose end of the loop.

Stretch Me Out: The Prusik Knot .
The French bowline cuff can also be secured to fixed points such as strategically placed wall hooks, or to any stable object whose design permits for the pleasures of sensual rope bondage, such as a chair or the uprights of a bed, with the Prusik knot.

Unlike the safety knot, the Prusik knot (see plate XI, page 171) ought never to be used directly on the body, as it will tighten when put under strain.

The Prusik knot provides for good control over the tension in the standing line, making for effective and dynamic restraints. The Prusik should never, ever be used directly on the body, because it tightens under strain.

Use the ends of the French bowline cuffs as the point of departure in learning how to tie the Prusik knot. Pass the free end of the French bowline cuff around your fixed stable point (for example, the upright of the bed). Pass the working end of the cord over the main line twice to form two loops (see *a* and *b* on plate XI, page 171). After the second loop has been made, the working end of the rope should be crossed over the engaged section of the working end of the cord that created the first loop then looped twice again in front of the first set of loops, beginning from under the main line (see *c*). Then pass the end of the cord inside the horizontal loop to complete the knot (see *d*). The end of the cord should now lie between the double loops that form the left and right sides of the Prusik knot.

Before tightening the knot, perfect its symmetry by pushing the loops together snugly down the taut main line (see *e*). When the Prusik is tight, it will lock down on the main line. When it is not, it can be slid up and down the main line. This is one of the Prusik's most notable assets—the tension on the cord can be increased and then released at will. The Prusik is particularly adapted for securing a consenting bottom in a spread-eagle position, as it allows the top not only to restrain the bottom but to gradually stretch them out ever so sweetly (always in accordance with the bottom's consent and physical limits).

Once the French bowline cuffs are secured to stable fixed points with the Prusik knot, the top should make sure that the cords always pass over the palms and not the backs of the bottom's hands, reducing the risk of putting their delicate articulations under strain or the pulse points under pressure. This safety measure has a fringe benefit: it gives the bottom a grip point that will render the struggles of his or her erotic captivity all the more dynamic!

Achieve Your Mission: Cord Extensions
An extension with a square knot can be created for a cord that is too short. This beautiful knot is created by twisting the ends of two separate ropes over each other, just as if you were getting ready to tie your shoe, but then, rather than making a bow, the cords are simply twisted over each other a second time. The trick lies in the direction in which these twists are made. Let's say you've created a French bowline cuff, but the standing line is not long enough to permit you to tie the bottom to a fixed point. You can extend the cord and achieve your mission by tying on another length of cord with the help of a square knot. Imagine that the ends of the two cords are labeled (or actually label them, if it's easier): the end used to make the French bowline cuff is "A," and the end of the extension is "B." The first twist should be made by passing A over B. The second and final twist should be made by twisting B over A. Pull the lines taut.

The square knot is ideal for joining two cords, as it tightens under strain. It therefore should never be used to secure binds directly on the body, as it cannot be released quickly.

The Sensual Embrace: Shibari and Compression
Certain forms of shibari serve to restrain the lover's sense of move-ment as well as provide the effects of compression. Those who enjoy wearing corsets are familiar with the erotic thrills of compression. Others have experienced its powers through wearing garments that are cut to hug every heavenly curve or are made of constrictive materials like latex, leather, or fabrics that cinch the silhouette such as Lycra or spandex. Tight-fitting clothing defines a body's underlying shape, creating an impact on the eye of the beholder. It also enhances body awareness, providing the wearer with an all-

over body hug that may rub him or her in all the right places!

Depending on how and where the cords are used, they may incite similar (but decidedly more acute) effects. The thighs, the chest, the breasts, and the genitals can be engaged in the hugging, rubbing, and constrictive embrace of the cords. The greater the surface areas of the body that are bound, the greater the overall effects will be—as long as the "no" zones are respected. Restriction and compression can combine for ecstatic results: The areas constricted by the cords become engorged with blood and grow even more sensitive to touch, while compression also induces a calming effect, facilitating the bottom's ability to truly abandon himself or herself to the sensual realm.

More Tantalizing Restraints
A basic shibari technique to restrain the wrists can also be used to restrain the legs, arms, and ankles, as well as tie the wrists to the ankles (see plate XII, page 172). Invite the bottom to put his or her hands together, pulse point to pulse point, either at the front or the back of the body. Use a doubled 8-foot-long (2.5-meter) cord, and wrap it around both wrists two or three times, keeping the binds symmetrical and even. The cords should not cross over each other but lie flat against each other and the skin. If the pulse points do not face and therefore protect each other, make sure the cords lie slightly above or below, not directly on, them. The last time the doubled cord is wrapped around the wrists, bring the working ends back to the front of the bind. Adjust the band of cord to ensure that the loop created by the bend at the middle of the cord is about 4 inches (10 centimeters) long and the resulting bind is symmetrical and harmonious.

Thread the working ends of the cords through the space between the wrists and wrap all of the cords that form the bind a couple of times, if not more, depending on the slack that needs to be taken up and the length of the standing lines.

The last time you pass the ends of the cords between the wrists, bring them back to the front of the bind and secure the restraint by tying a safety knot with the working cords and the loop. Arrange the knot and any remaining cord length in such a way that the bottom cannot execute a fast release on his or her own. This basic restraint is as effective as it is aesthetically pleasing to behold. Before commencing to tantalize your bound lover and/or proceeding to execute, for example, a lower-body bond, check again that the cords are not too tight.

Complete Control: The Kaiyaku Kani, or the Crab
The Kaikyaku Kani, or "the crab," is a two-phased restraint. First invite the bottom to sit or to lie on his or her back, bending the knees toward the chest. Using a doubled cord that is 25 to 30 feet long (8 to 9 meters), wrap the cord around a paired wrist and ankle, then pass the ends of the cord through the loop. Wrap the cords in the opposite direction three or four times, creating the bind. Make sure to leave a little bit of space between the ankle and the wrist. Ensure that the center loop is positioned in the middle of the bind, then thread the working ends of the cord through it.

Take up the slack in the cords by running the ends of the cord through the space between the ankle and the wrist; wrap the ends at least once, preferably twice, around all of the cords. The bottom should not be able to slip out of the restraint, but he or she must be able to move his or her wrists! Secure this phase of the restraint by tying an overhand knot at the front of the bind. Repeat the same restraint on the other wrist and ankle.

The second phase of the crab entails restraining the legs. Using the remaining length of the doubled cord, bind the lower portion of the calf and the thigh. Next, take up the slack and secure the bind by passing the working ends of the cords through the space between the cords and the crook of the knee. Terminate the bind with an overhand knot, and repeat the same restraint on the other side of the body.

If you are using long cords and come up with extra length, once the legs have been restrained, you may wish to cross the working lines from the right knee to the left side of the body, and vice versa, and terminate the crab by making a safety knot at the back. If the working lines are not long enough to do this, the same results can be achieved by adding two extra lengths of doubled cord to the knee restraints. The effects of the restraint can also be intensified by passing a cord around the *back* of the neck and securing the working ends to the left and right knee binds, which will pull the upper body forward.

Touch, Tease, and Squeeze: The Chest Harness
The chest harness (see plate XIII, page 221) can be used on its own, or in combination with a variety of restraints, including the crab. It provides a snug hug that instills in the bottom a unique sense of calm and security while providing the top with a grip point that will permit him or her to maneuver the bottom with ease from the seated position onto his or her back, rendering the genitals more accessible. The chest harness compresses the chest and lifts a female partner's breasts—not only a delectable sight to behold but also an irresistible invitation to touch, tease, and please!

When creating the chest harness, as with any other restraint on a standing bottom, the top should remain in a fixed position as much as possible. That is, rather than moving around the bottom, the top should have the bottom turn according to the demands of creating the restraint. This will avoid the bottom getting entangled in lengthy cords. It also reinforces the effects of the power shift and induces a euphoric sense of displacement in the bottom.

To create a basic chest harness, I recommend a doubled cord

that is 40 feet long (12 meters). Hold the loop at the center of the bottom's back, just below the shoulder blades, and have the bottom spin slowly; adjust the rope as it wraps around the area just beneath the breasts of a woman or the lower portion of a man's chest. Once the bottom comes twice in full circle, pass the ends of the rope through the center loop at the back. Making sure that the lines do not cross each other and that the bind is harmonious and symmetrical, pull the cords snugly against the bottom's skin. (When a bottom has breast implants, care should be taken that the cords aren't pulled too tightly.)

Then ask the bottom to spin in the opposite direction, so that the ropes can be wrapped directly over the upper area of the breasts or chest. The resulting bind should be the same width as the lower one. Repeated wrapping will make for a more supportive, constrictive chest harness. Once the bottom comes full circle for the last time, the ends of the rope should be passed through the center loop at the back once again. Make sure the bind is symmetrical before pulling the cords taut.

Holding the cords taut, move to the bottom's side and guide the cords over one of the shoulders and down the center of the chest, over the horizontal lines forming the front of the chest harness; the working ends are then threaded under the cords that form the base of the harness at the sternum. Next, bring them back up and over the lines that created the first "strap." This will result in an elegant drop-shaped loop at the center of the harness. Guide the cords over the opposite shoulder, thread them around the knot at the center of the back, and then give them a controlled but decisive tug to increase the tension on the harness. (This gesture will also remind the bottom of who is in control of his or her pleasure!) Secure the chest harness with an overhand or square knot. Finally, check in to make sure that the bottom is comfortable.

The harness will gradually increase the sensitivity of the breasts and the nipples. Like any form of bondage that constricts the thorax, it will also slightly reduce the natural expansion of the lungs and therefore the amount of air taken in. As the involuntary act of breathing verges toward a more voluntary and conscious act, the entire body will be called upon to adjust to the reduction of oxygen in the bloodstream. Those who practice yoga use a similar kind of breath control to instill a concentrated state of mind. The effects of the chest harness can lead a bound bottom toward similarly deep meditative states and heighten overall perceptions and awareness. The bound bottom may also experience pleasant sensations of drifting or weightlessness.

Intricate Ecstasy: Kinbaku, or the Unknotted Tortoise Shell
The effects of compression in combination with restraint can be executed in a traditional variation of kinbaku—the unknotted tortoise shell (see plate XVI, page 224). As complicated as this variation appears to be, it is actually surprisingly simple to do. Use your longest cord of 40 feet (12 meters), double it, and place the loop over the bottom's head. Without pulling the cords tight, pull the main lines toward the center of the bottom's chest and run them straight through the legs, along either side of the genitals. Bring the ends of the main lines up along the back and through the loop at the back of the neck.

Do not pull the cords snug. The creation of the unknotted tortoise shell will gradually take up the slack. If the cord is initially too snug, the binding cannot be nearly as intricate, and it risks becoming too constricting to be considered physically pleasing for the bottom. The more elaborate the restraint becomes, the more aesthetically moving it will be for both partners. With practice you will learn to calculate the amount of slack required to execute the tortoise shell to a T!

Now separate the working lines, run them under the bottom's

arms, then ask the bottom to spin so you have access to his or her front. Working from the top of the body downward, cross the main lines at the front of the body over each other, then thread the ends of the working lines over the vertical lines and pull them snug. This will create the first diamond shape, as well as the first horizontal line across the top of the chest. Continue working in this manner, crossing the vertical lines on the front of the body, then at back of the body, in accordance with the design that you wish to make.

As you proceed, the cords will tighten, and periodically check that those cords that lie on either side of the genitals do not cross over each other. When the upper-body tortoise shell is complete, tie it off at the back with a square knot. You may wish to rig a vibrator into the cords that come into contact with the genitals, which will cause all the cords to vibrate. If you have extra cord at the back of the harness, you may decide to use it to tie the bottom's wrists together behind his or her back using the basic shibari technique learned earlier in this chapter. Finish this bind with a safety knot.

Feel free to add extra lengths of cord in order to accomplish variations on the theme; your imagination is the limit as long as you respect the "no" zones.

Sweet Torture: The Cock Ring
One of my favorite restraints is an alternative to the cock ring (see plate VII, page 119). Using at least 6 feet (2 meters) of ¼-inch-diameter (6-millimeter) cord, double it, and then wrap it around the fully erect penis and the testicles. Thread the ends of the cord through the center loop, and tug for a snug fit. (Try not to snag your lover's pubic hair in the bindings.) Ensure that the bind is not too tight, then wrap the ropes in the opposite direction, at least two or three times, if not more. Terminate the bond by hitching the free ends of the ropes into the main lines, at the top or the

bottom of the bind, and tie them off with the simple overhand knot. The extra cord can be used as a leash or reins for your wild pony, or succumb to the temptation to crisscross the cords up your lover's engorged shaft. Pulling the ends ever so gently as you go will push his pleasure to celestial heights. Now that the vas deferens—and, therefore, the ejaculation reflex—are under delightful control, you can torture him with sweet ecstasy until he sees stars!

Euphoric Release
The way in which a bottom is released from the embrace of the cords, no matter where they are placed on the body, is as important to the positive outcome of the session as their skillful, harmonious application. When possible, the bottom should continue to move according to the top's instructions and refrain from touching the cords as they slip away from his or her body.

If the top prefers a bottom's release to be slow, the bottom's senses and breathing pattern will gradually readjust to a usual functioning state. If, on the other hand, the cords are released suddenly, the bottom will enjoy a sensory rush, a euphoric sense of liberation. Once all the cords have been removed, the bottom should be invited to relax and revel in the afterglow of the sensual rope bondage session.

CHAPTER 17

———o———

X MARKS THE SWEET SPOT:
EROTIC FLAGELLATION

I'm all for bringing back the birch, but only between consenting adults.

— Gore Vidal

FLAGELLATION MAY BE the most misinterpreted and controversial of all of the transcendental techniques in the Paradise Found Sexual Ceremony. Striking the body of another is regularly associated with violence, aggression, and punishment, and for good reason: whips, floggers, crops, and the like were designed not only to drive animals but to torture and punish human beings, so to uphold their use as a means of heightening degrees of sexual satisfaction is a challenging task.

You may have winced over an online depiction of a gory flagellation and wondered how and why anyone would submit himself or herself to such treatment in the name of pleasure. But when it comes to sex, the Internet thrives on extremes that draw attention, and therefore, business. In reality, erotic flagellation can be practiced as a means toward ecstatic sensations *without* causing physical or emotional harm—contrary to those sadomasochistic representations favored by the media, cinema, and the sex industry. When the tools are wielded skillfully—one can even say artistically—flagellation prompts a positive release and exchange of sexual energy.

No matter how "hard" or "soft" lovers play, physical abuse does not properly figure in a truly healthy sexual relationship. This cannot be reiterated enough: the needs, desires, and limits of the partner on the receiving end must be respected at all times. Good tops, whether they are sadists or not, only provide erotic flagellation in a safe, ritualized environment with full knowledge of and appreciation for the bottom's psychophysiological needs and the tools they are wielding. In the context of the Sexual Ceremony, the sole intent of a top is to transport the bottom, and consequentially himself or herself, toward higher dimensions in the sexual realm. Consent, like good intent, makes the difference between reality and ritual, between ecstasy and agony.

A look at the history of flagellation reveals the technique's once highly respected powers. Pre-Judeo-Christian cultures did not reserve the whip for purposes of punishment or torture alone; flagellation was used to purify and heal the body and absolve the spirit. Shamans from Siberia to Mesopotamia and from Africa to the Americas used flagellation in initiation rites of passage, and in many parts of the world the practice continues today. Ritualized whipping might still be used to avert evil spirits, ensure fertility, ease the pain of childbirth, or open a portal into the spiritual realm.

Pagan cults that worshipped the god Dionysus in Greece and Diana the Huntress in Rome practiced ritualized flagellation to induce euphoria and facilitate sexual transcendence. Even the Christian priesthood adopted flagellation—pagan practices for attaining heightened states of consciousness are often at the foundation of Christian rituals. However, unlike their pagan ancestors, these ascetic holy fathers practiced (and preached!) flagellation solely for the purpose of self-punishment. Ritual flagellation was performed by the faithful in private as well public ceremonies and even parades. Impure acts or thoughts were allegedly driven out of the spirit by the beatings. Those who enjoy erotic flagellation could conclude that this "punishment" was the means for ascetics to realize unfulfilled and denied sexual desires, as the effects of flagellation not only induce endorphin elation but also, for some individuals, provoke orgasm. Some aficionados of erotic flagellation actually prefer the pleasures of the whip to those of intercourse and penetration.

Corporal punishment was always the primary purpose of flagellation in Judeo-Christian cultures. However, during the period of the European Enlightenment, approximately 1650 through 1800, doctors began to prescribe the technique as a remedy for sluggish constitutions, to revive the senses, and as a cure for male impotency.

A STIMULATING SUBJECT

Flagellation's association with sexual pleasure was not fully recognized, and thus not officially condemned, until the end of the nineteenth century, when the medical community categorized erotic flagellation as deviant or "abnormal" sexual behavior. But this has never stopped people from seeking the pleasures of the whip! Erotic flagellation was considered to be a predominantly English tradition—even called by other Europeans "the English vice"—probably instigated by the once-accepted practice of corporal punishment of children in schools. Up through the 1950s, London was the city most renowned in Europe for accessible "spanking houses" and public "whipping clubs," where flagellation could be practiced openly, even as a group pleasure.

In reality, sexually mature adults who appreciate erotic flagellation come from all corners of the earth; rarely have these flagellation aficionados been chastised at home or school or been victims of other forms of abuse or violence. If you have longed to experience the exhilarating effects of spanking, whipping, or flogging but have refrained for fear of being labeled or hurt, now is the time to invite your partner to help you shed your shame, dissolve your fears, and make your fantasy a guiltless reality. Share *The Boudoir Bible* with your partner;

help him or her understand that your desire to experience erotic flagellation, either as top or bottom, is within the parameters of healthy sexual behavior.

Though most of the tools and techniques of erotic flagellation (see plate XV, see page 223) serve to stimulate specific areas of the body with precision, their psychophysiological impact is paradoxically all encompassing. The proficient provision of sensations with soft whips, floggers, riding crops, and similar instruments heightens the bottom's perceptive capacity and awakens his or her every sense. When purveyed skillfully by the top, in alternation with genital pleasures, flagellation prompts the blood to circulate readily throughout the entire body—not just to the areas that are directly stimulated. The sexual vibration mounts and begins to radiate from its source, charging the entire body with the erotic pulse. This makes the technique a wildly ecstatic and invigorating theme for any session, as well as a promising prelude to other ceremonial pleasures.

Novices to erotic flagellation should refrain from pushing limits—their own or anyone else's—before they have discovered what these limits are, which is only possible through practice. Skilled tops neither insist that the bottom submit unconditionally to his or her whip hand nor impose the more extreme forms of flagellation upon an occasional partner or novice.

As with the other transcendental techniques, this practice is an act of trust. Its bonding powers are strengthened by the top's impeccable degree of control (and good aim) but also through excellent communication skills, as elaborated in the chapter "Honor Each Other: Safety," a must-read before exploring flagellation.

THE "NO" ZONES AND "YES, YES, YES!" ZONES

Erotic flagellation demands a certain amount of anatomical understanding in order to be administered skillfully and, thus, safely.

The fleshy areas of the body will have a more positive, erotic response to flagellation, with the buttocks being the only area of the body that can be lovingly whipped, spanked, or flogged without posing any real risk of putting a bottom in danger. But before dwelling on the delights of the derrière, it's essential to know the parts of the body that should simply never be struck with anything other than a feather!

Like the "no" zones of sensual rope bondage, detailed in the chapter "Abandon Yourself: Erotic Restraints," the "no" zones for erotic flagellation (see plate IX, page 169) are those areas of the body where blood vessels lie close to the surface: the neck, the back of the knees, the crook of the elbows, the inner wrists, the armpits, the fine skin of the ankles, and the groin area. Striking these zones, no matter how lovingly, can be dangerous—so caress, tickle, and kiss, but don't whip!

The same rule applies to the entire circumference of the waist, no matter how fleshy it may be. All vital organs are vulnerable, so do not risk bruising the intestines, stomach, liver, or kidneys, which lie within the vulnerable waistline's soft walls. Also to be avoided are the areas where bones lie close to the surface: the shins, collarbone, the spinal column, the ribs, the fingers and toes, and the fragile tailbone—these areas will rarely incite an erotic response, and striking at bones can reap grave consequences. There are two unusual exceptions—the sternum and the sacrum, which will be explored in detail with the techniques of erotic cropping.

The face is also off-limits, but for one controversial exception: the slap. Certain lovers may enjoy the administration of a perfectly aimed and impeccably timed lust slap (done with the tips of the fingers, *not* the palm of the hand). The psychological impact of face slapping is more intense than the sensation itself. If your lover wishes to explore the psychophysiological effects of a carefully calculated lust slap, he or she should dare to ask for it, and your target must be the center of the fleshiest area of your wanton lover's cheek. Slapping any other zone of the face, including the ears, is dangerous. The timing of a slap is so crucial to its positive reception. I would recommend that this gesture be reserved for partners who enjoy its effects, and only if they simply adore each other and are both highly sexually aroused! These conditions are pertinent to the use of any instrument of erotic flagellation. Aside from the target of the careful hand, however, the head, the neck, and the face are always to be considered strictly off-limits . . . unless the bottom is invited to kiss a warm whip, crop, or flogger to express his or her gratitude!

The highly sensitive inner arms and the inner thighs, like the sides of the torso and the breasts, are very delicate areas of the body, and while not strictly off-limits during every form of flagellation, they need to be approached with caution. The palms of the hands and soles of the feet are highly charged with nerve endings and may be sweetly cropped or whipped to delight, but high-impact blows are to be avoided. The *Kama Sutra* encourages lovers to flagellate the muscular areas of the shoulders, the upper back, the hips, and the torso, as well as the buttocks. When striking these areas of the body, the top's aim must be precise enough to strike at the shoulder muscles and not the shoulder blades; the upper back and the muscles that sustain the spine but not the waist or the spinal column itself; the hips but not the hip bones; and the muscles of the upper chest but not the breasts, collarbone, or neck.

Until the top is a skilled master of the wielded tool, he or she will want to concentrate most of the attention on the bottom's bottom—not only the safest place to administer any form of erotic flagellation but, for many, the most erogenous spot to receive such attentions. As the muscles of the buttocks are the largest in the body, they are more tolerant to direct, intense contact.

Not to be ignored is that lower portion of the buttocks that meets the backs of the legs, known as "the sweet spot" (see plate

XIV, page 222). This area contains a great number of nerve endings, some of which are connected to the glands of the genitals, both the penis and the clitoris. Stimulating the sweet spot is therefore an indirect means of stimulating the genitals, which explains why erotic flagellation can inspire heightened sexual arousal as well as orgasm.

The buttocks may be tantalized by every tool and technique available to inspired lovers, but there is nothing that can compare to the invigorating dance of the whip hand and other tools. But before the top commences to "cherry" the well-aroused bottom's cheeks, locate the bottom's sacrum—the triangular bone that lies at the base of the spine. From there, run the fingers down to the coccyx, or the tailbone. This tapered end of the spinal cord is fragile enough to break under the impact of a poorly delivered stroke and should never be struck.

PRIME POSITIONS TO BETTER THE PLEASURE

Tops must make certain that the bottom is in a stable position, one that will permit him or her to respond, without injury, to the impact of every stroke and strike. If sensations are to be administered for a psychological response—for example, in the context of role-play that might explore ritualized humiliation—the bottom may be put into a position that reflects the motivation for the spank, whip, or flog. The interrelation of the top's and the bottom's bodies will be determined not only by the tool or technique but also by the session's encompassing motivation.

Even though the tools and techniques of erotic flagellation automatically reinforce the roles of top and bottom, not everyone is ready to delve into the psychology of subservience. Bottoms who are seeking only a sensory experience are not likely to appreciate being pulled over the top's knee like a naughty child. Nor will this bottom feel comfortable in the classic "schoolboy" position: bending over at the waist to grasp the ankles. (Note that this position compromises the bottom's balance, and it should never be used when high-impact sensations are in store.) Lovers who do not wish to explore the deeper psychological effects of erotic flagellation may prefer less theatrical positions: if you are such a bottom, stand and brace yourself with your hands against a wall, with your feet about shoulders' width apart, or bend over a sturdy piece of furniture or go down on all fours. Bent positions provide perfect access to the buttocks as well as to the ever-enchanting genitals. They also stretch the skin, bringing nerve endings and blood vessels closer to the surface, therefore enhancing sensitivity.

When the bottom is a man, the top must be extremely careful to avoid striking his testicles. The bottom may cover his "family jewels" with a hand if they is not restrained. The top can likewise give protection with his or her hand that is not employed, but this has the disadvantage of limiting agility and control. To keep his testicles out of harm's way, the bottom might wear a thong (although not everyone will appreciate that aesthetic). If the top is skilled in the art of cock-and-ball bondage and the bottom enjoys its effects, the penis as well as the testicles can be bound in such a manner as to be drawn out of danger, a creative solution that can be achieved by combining the techniques of sensual cock-and-ball rope bondage and basic kinbaku, described in the section on sensual rope bondage in the chapter "Abandon Yourself: Erotic Restraints." Another solution is to have the male bottom close or cross his legs.

Male or female, if the bottom is standing, care must be taken so that the bottom does not lose balance. If he or she is standing with feet together, there must be a place to brace against the impact of each strike or stroke. The bottom's feet should never be bound together unless his or her upper body is fully supported. In general, less risky positions, such as on all fours, are the best place to start experimenting. Over time and with experience, lovers will discover the most comfortable and convenient positions. The partner who is providing sensations should feel free to help his or her bottom find a balanced position—thus reinforcing the role of the top, which the receptive bottom won't mind a bit. Novice tops should confine their attention to the buttocks only and refrain from using any tools other than their hands; that is, they should experiment first with spanking.

A PROPER WARM-UP: SPANKING

Hand spanking provides for an intimate exchange between partners and is an excellent initiation into the psychophysiological effects of flagellation. Until the 1950s, the first direct contact that a newborn baby had with another human being, upon his or her entry into the world, was a perfectly calculated spank on the buttocks by the firm hand of the obstetrician. This caused the baby to cry out of surprise (not pain), clearing the lungs of fluids and filling them with air. Modern hospitals now employ a device that suctions fluids from the baby's mouth, so a machine has replaced the primal spank.

Erotic spanking has a similar capacity to jump-start both the body and mind, sending a seemingly desensitized or sluggish person into an erotic whirl. The manually administered spank has the unique advantage of being easy to combine with other forms of stimulation, including penetration—as long as both partners are well aroused. Any technique that opens the doors to the sexual dimension is a good prelude to erotic flagellation, as a proper warm-up is essential. As the ceremony evolves, the ideal moment for an erotic spank will arise; a good top will know how and when to take advantage—and the aroused bottom could also beg for it, to the top's delight.

To reduce the stinging impact of each loving strike on the top's hand (as well as the bottom's bottom), the purveyor should cup his or her hand, holding the fingers firmly together. Thin, unlined leather gloves or latex gloves can be worn to keep that distinct sting that spanking prompts from radiating into the hands of the purveyor of the exhilarating pleasures. Gloves, also considered fine erotic accessories by many, bring exciting acoustic effects to the session. So don't forget to respect those not taking part in your ceremonial pleasures—make sure that the room is soundproofed. Spanking makes a delightful noise!

Start the spanking session by "smoothing out" the bottom's buttocks with your hands. Then caress, squeeze, and tantalize the delectable flesh of these nether regions to get a feeling for their layout. This preparatory contact reinforces the intimate bond and prepares both bottom and top mentally as well as physically. Once every rise and fall, dip and ripple of the bottom's contours have been lovingly assessed, the spanking may commence.

Light, fleeting taps and the occasional squeeze get the session rolling. The timing of your first real strike must be exactly right. As the bottom eases into the sensations, move on again with light taps, then with more calculated strokes, and possibly a few decisive strikes. A deft, slapping gesture, the hand leaving the bottom's buttocks the instant after contact, reduces both the impact of the spank and the risk of generating oversensitivity. Spank the buttocks with rhythmic strokes with an upward, "lifting" gesture.

Between each more intense spank, intersperse soft and subtle sensations, for example a shower of reassuring caresses and some genital attentions, too. This will avoid sensory overload in your bottom and allow sexual tension to mount gradually. Take your time. Alternating degrees of intensity and the areas of contact will keep the experience from becoming predictable, enhancing the psychological impact of the ritual. When the bottom begs for more, the top may choose to give him or her less, and vice versa. The rhythm of the session should be maintained through such artful variations as balancing the number of strikes made on the left and the right sides of the body, always returning to stimulating the genitals. Introducing a light, feathery tool mid-session will be perceived as a gracious gesture and an enlightening sexual experience!

As you progressively stimulate the bottom, his or her bloodstream will receive a steady flow of endorphins. Day-to-day worries, along with any preconception of what "pain" might be, will dissolve in deep pleasure. Where the mind goes, the body follows—so novice tops should not be surprised when their lovers beseech them for more intense strikes. Don't push the limits established before the ceremony began. The bottom's threshold for pain will naturally increase because endorphins are natural painkillers, so novice or skilled, the top must always proceed with caution, keeping his or her exhilarated flagellant under close observation at all times.

TEN GOOD STRIKES

Lovers who intend not only to test but also push limits should implement the "gauge of good strikes." This means that before the session begins, both top and bottom define the maximum number of "good" strikes that may be administered before the session's end. Good strikes are those that are just intense enough to reach or, at the most, gingerly push the bottom's limits—and not surpass them. It will be the bottom's responsibility to voice each good strike out loud; ten good strikes are normally enough to bring the bottom to his or her limit.

By essentially putting the bottom in control, the "gauge of good strikes" helps to guarantee the ritual's harmonious evolution and prevents the error of the bottom's limits being overstepped. When the bottom says "one," the top understands this as the first good strike, and thereby gauges the intensity for each strike following. Good strikes incite a wild rush of sexual energy, which further releases endorphins. The strikes should fall first on one side of the body, then on the other, intermingled with a shower of ethereal, cooling caresses and sumptuous genital attentions. The more the top is in control of all of his or her generous resources, the more the bottom will surrender to the sensual realm and the more enduring and exhilarating the session will be for both partners.

While good strikes may be accompanied with an involuntary flinch, if the bottom resists or recoils from the top's attentions, the top should interpret the reaction as an indication that he or she has surpassed the bottom's limits. The bottom should be able to trust that the top will stop and smooth his or her rosy, smarting soul with more tender, loving care. If a bottom's limits have been involuntarily surpassed, genital pleasures are the most thrilling way for the top to say, "Sorry, baby."

Once the bottom has been coaxed back into a relaxed, receptive state of mind, the session of erotic flagellation may be resumed. But it's the bottoms call to do so—and the bottom's wish is the top's command. If the top insists upon administering sensations that are not in accord with the bottom's needs, desires, and limits, it is the bottom's right to bring the ceremony to an end.

Overzealous, forceful, fleeting, and unexpected blows that surpass the bottom's psychophysiological limits—prompting the bottom to call out the good strikes in a hurried sequence, use the safe word "red," or protect himself or herself from blows—are unacceptable. The infliction of real pain—that is, beyond the pain threshold of the bottom, or outside the context of consensual, loving agreement—has absolutely nothing to do with the philosophy of *The Boudoir Bible*.

When the ceremony has progressed harmoniously, the top will notice the bottom's skin beginning to take on a rosy color as blood rushes to the skin's surface; it will also be warm if not hot to the touch. Such transformations herald the transmission of energy and are clear signals that the areas are now more sensitive. This is one reason why the intensity of a strike, after the first "good strike," does not have to be increased in order to make an impact. As the top takes care to monitor the intensity of each strike, so endorphin elation in the bottom transforms what might otherwise be interpreted as pain into a rush of pleasurably intense and possibly transcendental sensations.

When the bottom voices "ten," the end of the flagellation is nigh, and the ceremony now takes on new focus. The top may soothe the bottom's hot, rosy cheeks one last time with sweet, gracious caresses. Engaging in genitally oriented pleasures highlights the positive effects of spanking or other erotic flagellations. Orgasms experienced shortly after a flagellation session bring an entirely new meaning to the word "pleasure."

NOT YOUR HEADMASTER'S SPANKING BOARDS!

Spanking can be done with other implements, too. Many Anglo-Saxons will recall the days when a board, paddle, or cane was an acceptable means to punish schoolchildren. I will never forget the sight of the board that hung on the wall behind the headmaster's imposing desk at my school. It was made of solid oak, its handle branded with the school's mascot—a growling bulldog—and it was feared. Those who had the misfortune to taste its bite did not wish to do so twice.

But unless you and your partner are bona fide sadomasochists, cumbersome spanking boards, heavy paddles, and canes are next to impossible to use lovingly. For the purpose of the Paradise Found Sexual Ceremony, partners are therefore encouraged to seek out the lighter paddles designed explicitly for erotic spanking (see plate XIV, page 222). Paddles have never been more available in a wider variety of materials, shapes, and sizes than they are today. Many of these instruments can be wielded with a lighter hand, but all of them should be used with tapping gestures at the start, not strikes. As the bottom warms up and grows increasingly aroused, he or she may crave more intense contact. Whether made of leather, wood, or other materials, light paddles are easy to control, so the top is not likely to surpass the bottom's limits. But a word of warning: with overuse, even light paddles can inflict injurious sensations. If these are incurred repeatedly, session after session, damage to nerve endings and blood vessels may result—an unfortunate condition called "leather butt" in BDSM jargon, which is a desensitization of the sweet spot. And that is a consequence that no lover would want to inflict upon another!

The strap is usually composed of one or two thick leather flaps or straps. Its impact will depend on its weight and the kind of leather from which it is made—the heavier and less supple the hide, the more the strap must be handled with care. The sensations from light straps can be compared to those provided with the hand. Straps further provide an acoustical thrill, even when used in moderation— a sound that heightens the psychological impact of the ceremony for both top and bottom. Some of you may have a memory of your father's belt chastising your tender hindquarters, not to mention your burgeoning psyche. But the aim of the top, in the context of the Sexual Ceremony, is always to provide pulsating, erotic pleasure, not distress and pain!

A FLICK OF THE WRIST: WHIPS, CROPS, FLOGGERS, AND CATS

Once consenting lovers have explored the powers and pleasures of erotic spanking to their satisfaction, they may wish to explore whips. The term "whip" is commonly used to define a wide variety of instruments—some designed to control animals, others to punish human beings, and yet others fashioned specifically for erotic flagellation.

The cat, the riding crop, the flogger, and the horsetail whip especially are hailed for their capacity to provide for a full-body experience, prompting circulation, increasing overall sensitivity, and permitting lovers to engage in lengthy rituals. Contrary to their menacing appearance, these instruments actually incite sensual sensations that range from feathery to moderate to intense. When used skillfully and in harmony with the bottom's limits, they may inspire a wide range of pleasures without necessarily inspiring any threshold of pain. The basic guidelines for the safe use of whips are essentially the same as those pertaining to spanking. New rules will arise in light of the fact that these tools present an inestimable advantage: they may pleasure areas other than the buttocks.

Like the paddle and the strap, the cat, crop, flogger, and horsetail whips should also be considered extensions of the hand. The gesture that sets them into action should come from the wrist, not the arm. Novices can first practice the dance of the whip on an inanimate object, perfecting the aim and acquiring that distinctive flick of the wrist. Compact pillows are the best target—if covered in leather, all the better!

Let's say you have acquired good control and a sexy rhythm, and that you have perfected your aim; nevertheless, before targeting your lover's bottom, test the new tool on your own naked skin. The self-administration of sensations will not be perceived as acutely as any laid on by another, but testing your new whips, cats, crops, and floggers on your forearm, the muscular area of the outer thighs, and, when possible, on the buttocks will enlighten you as to the sensational potential of the tool.

Those lovers who enjoyed being spanked can look forward to the possibility of being cropped, flogged, or carefully whipped; all such sensations are quite different from a spank.

The bottom can be in a few positions that are conducive to such pleasures: lying face down, on all fours, standing in a stable position, or safely restrained. These positions permit the top to move around the body freely in a natural, harmonious manner; a top can think of leading a three-way dance between the bottom, the tool in hand, and himself or herself. The top may administer brisk taps, moderate strokes, and at the maximum a few harder strikes, unless the bottom actually prefers more intense sensations.

Genteel Seduction

Lovers have probably appreciated the powers of the riding crop, beyond its equestrian function, ever since it was invented. Traditionally made of cane covered with woven leather strips, crops are now usually composed of a flexible shaft made of fiberglass covered with woven leather strips or a synthetic fabric mesh. The riding crop terminates in a leather tongue called a popper, lash, or quirt, depending on its form.

In the context of the Paradise Found Sexual Ceremony, the more genteel nature of those crops that terminate with a flat leather tongue, or popper, finds their place. If, when shopping for your crop, you are seduced by one made in pastel leather, or with a handle encrusted with rhinestones rather than a more menacing, studded, black leather model—go for it! But keep in mind that these fashionable crops, as feminine and glamorous as they seem to be, are as potent as those with a more hardcore aesthetic.

Crops are used to sensitize very precise areas of the body with very targeted strikes, charging the bottom's body with tingling delight. Unless tops are skilled at the art of erotic cropping, attentions should be confined to the buttocks, the upper thighs, and the sides of the hips. These areas may be stimulated with the popper as well as with the shaft of the crop, but in the latter case, the top must exercise greater self–control. The shaft of the crop is capable of inflicting extreme sensations (and welts), similar to those evoked by canes. Because of the cane's "extreme" potential to provide sensations as well as painful bruises and marks, I have excluded the cane from the Paradise Found repertoire—with all due respect for those who need pain in order to experience pleasure.

The muscular areas of the upper arms, the shoulders, and the muscles that support the spinal column, like the backs of the legs, will all respond ecstatically to the crop's leather tongue. The soles of the feet can also be carefully cropped, but the delicate skin in the crook of the knees ought never be struck.

The Sacred Charge
While cropping the waistline is strictly forbidden, skilled tops may tantalize the sacrum, which lies at the base of the spine. The sciatic nerve and other sacral nerves, some of which terminate in the genitals, pass through the bone's triangular structure. This connectivity helps explain why it responds well to stimulation, and how this "sacred" bone was so named.

We have the bone's description first from the Greeks, *hieron osteon*, meaning "holy bone." Translated into the Latin *sacer*, or "holy", our sacred sacrum has since been assumed by many cultures to be the source of humankind's procreative powers. Shamans from Mesoamerica to Siberia considered the sacrum to be a cosmic portal to and from the spiritual dimension. The sacrum is formed by the fusion of six vertebrae—a developmental process that does not reach completion until adults are approximately twenty-six years of age. While stimulating the sacrum ever so carefully with the crop, avoid striking the fragile tailbone. The sacrum may also be deeply massaged. This charges the genitals with an ecstatic pulse of energy.

The only other bone that may be the object of flagellatory stimulation is the sternum, the flat bone that lies at the center of the chest. The sternum acts as the heart's protective shield and braces the ribcage. The *Kama Sutra* suggests that lovers tap the sternum to elicit sexual energy. Within the Paradise Found Sexual Ceremony, it can be approached, not by striking, but with very soft, light taps of the crop's leather tongue. If the bottom is not comfortable with this sensation, similarly positive effects may be obtained, as with the sacrum, by massaging the area with the fingertips.

Specialists in Indian Ayurvedic medicine consider the sternum to be the location of the heart chakra. To open this center of human compassion, they practice specific disciplines. The result is a putting aside of the ego, allowing love to enter the spirit, and feeling the desire to be of service to others. If the top might effect this response in the bottom, it is an ideal state for both of them to be in!

Yet it must be understood that striking the sternum is dangerous. The soft tip of the riding crop is the only instrument of erotic flagellation that will provide a skilled top with enough precision to safely stimulate this area. Though crops permit for a greater degree of control than other whips, their use on the front of the body should be limited to the sternum, the inner and outer thighs, and the muscular zones of the upper torso. Cropping the neck or face, the ribs, breasts, or collarbone verges on punishment and is dangerous. The nipples may be teased to attention with the very tip of the crop, but as with the genitals, these vulnerable zones should not be struck. Tickle and tease only; these delights will more than suffice.

Good Medicine
No matter the genre of whip, the longer its lashes, the more difficult it will be to control. The lashes of long whips, floggers, and cats range in length from approximately 12 inches to 20 inches (30 to 50 centimeters), excluding the handle. If the lashes correspond more or less to the length of the forearm of the person using it, he or she will feel more in control of the tool. To determine the length best for you, measure from the crease of the elbow to the tip of the middle finger. Long whips are best for back stimulation, while shorter whips, which range from 6 to 10 inches (15 to 25 centimeters), excluding the handle, work well for frontal stimulation. Short

floggers make a slighter impact and provide the degree of control necessary to avoid striking the neck, face, or eyes with its lashes. Novice tops should train with the shorter version, which are less likely to "wrap," strike off the target, or "come back," giving the novice a taste of the good medicine they are dosing out!

The horsetail whip is the most versatile of the instruments of erotic flagellation (see plate XX, page 278). In the context of the tickle ritual, its use makes for a wonderfully smooth transition from a bout of erotic tickling to one of flagellation, or vice versa. When used to its full potential, it provides for a distinctly pleasant and invigorating sting that flushes fresh, oxygenated blood throughout the bottom's system. Such sensations heighten the bottom's overall sensory awareness, enhance his or receptivity, and, as with any flagellation performed skillfully, leave the bottom feeling both physically and mentally purified.

The horsetail whip is an excellent prelude to any other form of contact. As it may be used to stimulate large surfaces areas of the body without provoking sensory overload, it is particularly adapted to lengthy sessions. The sound that the horsetail whip makes is also low impact, more of a *swish* or *swoosh* than the *slap*, *crack*, and *clap* of other flagellators, making it a discreet travel accessory.

Like any long whip or flogger, the horsetail whip may be used while the bottom is lying down, in a relaxed position. If the bottom is lying on his or her back, the eyes should be protected with a blindfold or, for example, the edge of the bedsheet. When the bottom is lying on his or her stomach, he or she should likewise cover the eyes or keep the head in a frontal position, with eyes closed, while the upper area of the back is being flagellated.

Using the horsetail whip with forceful strikes is the most common mistake the inexperienced top makes. Graceful sweeps (much like those that horses make with their tails) suffice. Do not attempt to strike with greater impact with the horsetail whip—the ends of the hairs can break off and become embedded in the bottom's skin.

Removing them one by one, with tweezers, from your now highly sensitized bottom's skin is tedious and anything but erotic.

The horsetail whip is unique in that there is no area of the body, other than the face and neck, that it cannot tantalize to a warm, tingling glow. If your bottom consents, you can use the horsetail whip to softly stroke the genitals, nipples, and breasts. You may also stroke the area of the waistline, otherwise off-limits during other erotic flagellations, but note that this area of the body does not usually incite an erotic response. The longer horsetail whip is best used to stimulate the back of the body; other lengths are more all-purpose.

Sweet Sensations

Once a warm, tingling glow envelops the bottom's body, he or she may crave more direct and intense forms of contact. The rhythm of the session can be gradually intensified through the implementation of soft floggers (see plate XV, page 223). In contradiction to their menacing appearance, soft floggers are unable to inflict sensations that can be described as seriously painful, even when used to their full potential. Imagine what it would feel like to have one hundred soft, minuscule hands slapping your backside, in rhythmic unison, with all their tiny might, and you have a pretty good idea of the impact that soft floggers make. Were it not for the vicious slapping sound that each strike makes when the soft lashes come into contact with bare skin, professional masseurs would probably adopt soft floggers. The flogger's skillful use is an excellent alternative to the erotic massage, but its effects are more invigorating.

The softer the flogger, the sweeter the sensations it will provide. Those composed of flat, thin strips of supple leather, rubber, suede, or deer hide of approximately ⅜ inch (1 centimeter) in width provide for deep, invigorating sensations. Floggers made of stiff hide or other rough materials provide extreme sensations and can even break the skin if wielded with force; their use is therefore not in alignment with the philosophy of *The Boudoir Bible.*

Areas with more muscle mass, like the buttocks, are best suited to experience the sensations that arise from erotic flagellation. The front of the body, *excluding the waistline,* can be approached, but only with short floggers and in moderation. Drag the flogger sweetly over the "no" zones, and even the entire body from time to time. Though floggers may be used while the bottom is lying down, positions that allow the bottom to brace his or her body and respond more effectively to the deep thud that each stroke will make is best, especially if the tool is going to be used to its full potential.

Some men and women appreciate the effects of their genitals being gently flogged. When the bottom is a man, strokes must be made with light, downward sweeps. Flogging the testicles with upward strokes, no matter how gently, is likely to make him very nervous. But some men very much enjoy the "edge play" of this stimulation. Use instruments that do not lash the skin, and lay it on very lightly. Otherwise the top may inflict one of the greatest pains known to mankind! The same rule applies to the flogging of the female genitals—go gently. If you are not skilled in the use of the flogger, concentrate your attention only upon the backside of your partner's body.

A Gentler Breed
Unlike the cat-o'-nine-tails (familiar to many from depictions of BDSM flagellation), erotically charged cats are cats of a gentler breed, composed of multiple lashes of supple, non-braided leather, suede, rubber, or cotton. They can inflict pain if used without control, but in the context of the Sexual Ceremony, they are used with restraint and with the aim to gradually charge the body with the sexual vibration. Cats made of cotton are capable of provoking sensations as intense as those made by leather or rubber, so do

not be fooled by their seeming flaccidity. Suede cats may be harder to come by, but they are by far the sweetest race of all of the cats. Be aware, however, that if these are used without a degree of restraint, they may leave telltale signs behind, as with any other thin-lashed variety of whip.

When used with moderation, cats raise a radiant glow on the bottom's skin. The distinct stinging sensations that the cat can evoke will lead to heightened states of sensory arousal. Compare these sensations to those inspired by the instrument called "the birch," or *vihta*, of Finland. It is composed of bundles of young, soft, leafy birch branches, with a handle created by tying the ends together with twine. Birches can also be made from the relatively soft branches of other trees, such as cedar or poplar. The vihta is traditionally used in steam saunas to excite a pleasant "smart" that enhances circulation, opens the pores, and helps the body expel toxins. The association of birching with health and hygiene renders the technique probably the most openly accepted form of flagellation, especially in Scandinavian countries, where the steam sauna is essentially a cultural affair. The vihta must not be confused with the birching rod, used for corporal punishment in nineteenth-century England. Unlike the softer, leafy twigs of the vihta, the twigs of the birching rod are stripped of their leaves with the intent to inflict harsh pain and leave enduring and anything but endearing marks.

When trying out the impact of any new cat, novice bottoms may wish to keep their "knickers" on to protect against undue pain. Safe words, the gauge of "good strikes," and lovers' checking in with each other frequently are all pertinent to the positive outcome of cat rituals. Refer to the chapter "Honor Each Other: Safety" to review the conditions for the proper use and reception of the instruments of desire.

As with all instruments of erotic flagellation, the dance of the cat demands controlled and concise flicks of the wrist. Cats may be used to sensitize not only the buttocks but also the back of the thighs, the sides of the hips, the upper back, and the muscles that support the spine. The feet may also be whipped, but only very mildly. Cats may also be used to tickle the nipples and the genitals to attention. Don't forget to drag the fine lashes of the cat over the bottom's skin from time to time, as a caressing reminder that you care.

Two whips that cannot be used, beyond a purely symbolic purpose, in the temple of erotic loving are the aforementioned cat-o'-nine-tails and its distant cousin, the single-tail bullwhip. When used to their full potential, these whips can be extremely "mean." The cat-o'-nine tails originally had the specific purpose of punishing human beings. The bullwhip, also called the stock whip, was designed to drive and control livestock—a recalcitrant bull, in particular. The cat-o'-nine tails is constructed of nine finely braided thongs that are each knotted at the striking end. This instrument leaves stripes resembling the claw marks of a tiger and feeling that just as acute, deep, and lasting! The cat-o'-nine tails once served to administer corporal punishment in such institutions as the British royal navy and was called "the captain's daughter." Unless you are a bona fide masochist who neither minds being marked nor suffering serious wounds, do not allow the cat-o'-nine tails to come anywhere near your naked skin.

Likewise, the bullwhip cannot be used to its full potential without inflicting serious pain. Though both cat-o'-nine tails and bullwhips may serve as symbols of sexual dominance, within the Sexual Ceremony they are best employed only for their psychological impact, for example, in role-play rituals involving aggression or punishment. Otherwise, they are not recommended beyond a tickle or a visual "tease."

The skilled top, sadistic or not, like a skilled cowboy, never cracks a bullwhip on the flesh of a human being (or animal, for that matter). The distinct *crack* of the bullwhip occurs because the tip is moving faster than the speed of sound, creating a sonic boom. It is, in fact, the sound of the whip cracking that controls the cattle, not its cutting edge against their hides.

For tops with an exhibitionistic leaning, learning to master the crack of the bullwhip with the help of a skilled master can be great fun! There are even organized competitions in this skill. But unless you intend to work at the circus, learn to crack stock whips that range in length from 3 to 10 feet (1 to 3 meters). They are easier to control and less likely to "come back" on the trainee. Bullwhips should only be used in wide-open spaces.

SUPPLE AND READY TO PLEASE: CARE OF TOOLS

All instruments of erotic flagellation must be washed and disinfected regularly. Those made of wood, rubber, cotton, and leather can be cleansed with soap and warm water and swathed with disinfectant wipes. Tools made of wood or leather should not be allowed to absorb water. Those made of wood should be waxed (with chemical-free beeswax only), while those made of leather may best be treated with mink oil or other natural leather conditioner. Polish any applied oils or waxes to a sheen with a soft cloth. Keep wood oiled and leather supple and ready to please.

As you prepare the temple for a ritual that will include erotic flagellation, your selection of whips, cats, crops, or floggers should be set out at hand's reach. Include other instruments of desire to be used alternately, anticipating softer, more sensual intervals of both genital and extra-genital stimulation. These may be the likes of an ostrich feather tickler, a blindfold, erotic restraints, vibrators, dilettos, and gloves. Finally, come to your temple with a calm, cool, and concentrated mind, prepared to soar!

Lovers who appreciate ritualized erotic flagellation hail its power to test or push their sensory limits and intensify the sense of weightlessness, flying, and floating inherent to lovemaking. Tops who learn to prompt the steady flux of their bottom's natural love drug will instigate deeply satisfying rituals, and the invigorating effects—which have also been described as sexually exhilarating, physically aligning, and even spiritually enlightening—will endure long after the ceremony ends. When administered *ad arte*, erotic flagellation induces a lucid, focused, trancelike state of mind in both the provider and the receiver. The harmonious progression of the Paradise Found Sexual Ceremony via these radically heightened degrees of sexual satisfaction permits lovers to transcend the confines of physical space and leave the world behind in their own personal Paradise.

CHAPTER 18

———o———

BACK TO REALITY:
COMING DOWN

For pleasure has no relish unless we share it.

— Virginia Woolf, "Montaigne"

THE MANNER in which partners descend from the transcendental dimensions of the sexual realm—the return to reality—is as relevant to the positive outcome of the ceremony as their ascent to Paradise. Taking the time together to come down from the inebriating effects of endorphin elation reinforces the physical and emotional benefits of extended, ritualized playtime. The longer and more intense the journey, the longer it will take for the effects of the body's "love drug" to subside.

The Sexual Ceremony's skillful elaboration unveils the depths of the inner spirit; as it closes, some lovers will feel the need to revel in the luxury of silence. Others may wish to talk, not necessarily about the ritual itself, but about general topics. This is perfectly natural, but until the ceremony is completely over, continue to refrain from broaching subjects that could allow reality to invade the ritual dimension.

It is also probable that you will both be inclined to wrap your arms around each other and take a nap. Plummeting into deep sleep is the most natural response to an exhilarating round of Paradise Found. When you do eventually rise, you are likely to be very hungry. If you opt to terminate your return to reality over a restaurant dinner, beyond the confines of the temple walls, take a shower or a bath together to regenerate your energy. Keep in mind that interrelating with anyone who was not part of your journey may feel slightly awkward until the effects of endorphin elation have completely subsided.

Neither partner should abandon the ceremonial space abruptly or without forewarning; it will break the magic spell of the sacred moment. It can even incite negative cathartic reactions in the partner left alone in the vortex of energy that you generated together.

If the time frame that you have carved out of a busy schedule is limited, and you or your partner are obliged to exit the temple separately or at a predetermined hour, arrange this in advance. An alarm can be set at least thirty minutes before the ceremony must come to an end. In the case that partners intend to engage in techniques like bondage and flagellation that prompt endorphins more readily into the bloodstream, the intensity of the session should be regulated accordingly. Exploring and pushing sexual boundaries to more intense degrees simply requires more time dedicated to ceremonial endeavors.

Coming down from the effects of rituals that have endured a full day or more can leave lovers feeling slightly bemused and befuddled. Push on through the day, eat light meals, and drink plenty of water. As body and brain resume "normal" functioning, these sensations will subside. Partners who do not live together should make a point to contact each other the following day, just to make sure that each is as happy and well, physically, emotionally, and spiritually, as both were when going separate ways. This may also be the perfect occasion to set the date for your next journey to Paradise.

AFTERWORD

——————o——————

BEYOND THE BOUDOIR

If you love love, look for yourself.

— Rumi

THE ART OF LOVING, like the art of living, is founded on self-love—the ripe fruit of self-knowledge, understanding, and acceptance; it is as essential to our capacity to experience deep sexual satisfaction as it is to our harmonious evolution both as individuals and as a society.

To know, accept, and love ourselves is fundamental to our capacity to know, accept, and love others. The better we get to know ourselves, the more likely we are to "rise" in love with our partners, rather than "fall" in love. To rise in love is to love creatively and freely; it is to love yourself as much as the one you love.

The Paradise Found Sexual Ceremony gives us the opportunity to love creatively and freely and, in the process, construct more profound, positive, and holistic relationships. It is an ecstatic meditation whose benefits—an antidote to the fleeting gratification of "fast," predominantly genitally oriented sex—lead to the attainment of deep sexual satisfaction. It inspires lovers to breathe into and focus their intent, to bring the sacred back into everyday life, and to explore the universe that is the body through sexual pleasure. The result of these loving actions will reverberate in more ways than one can imagine!

By engaging in such a meditation, we take responsibility for our pleasure and make it a priority. This nourishes our imagination, leading us to love in more original, adventurous, and deeply meaningful ways. Nourished by Eros, a daring and nonjudgmental imagination is the fountainhead of life, love, and sex. By charging the creative spirit, Eros keeps the heart and mind wide open and ready to explore, test, and stretch boundaries. The creative mind, with a passion for the freedom to please and to be pleased, does not restrict itself to predefined territories but rather maintains that healthy sense of liberty and adventure that allows us to surpass the limitations of categories, social conditioning, and convention and discover new dimensions of sexual satisfaction.

Ceremonial partners who feed their creative spirits and nourish their imaginations with experimentation, adventure, and invention find themselves on the very path that leads toward new—and possibly transcendental—sexual horizons. *The Boudoir Bible* is a call to these creative paths and an invitation to embrace the vulnerability that is inherent to the sexual bond and to the luxury of love.

May the Paradise Found Sexual Ceremony lead you and yours toward a life filled with greater and more all-encompassing pleasure, the key to the cultivation of deeper, more solid, and enduring intimate bonds—the foundation of sexual satisfaction and well-being. The personal transformations that the skillful elaboration of the Sexual Ceremony incite will thrust open doors to a more adventurous, exquisite, and fulfilling life—both in and beyond the boudoir.

BIBLIOGRAPHY

―――――○―――――

Albert, Nicole G. *Saphisme et décadence*. Paris: Editions de la Martinière, 2005.

Angier, Natalie. *Woman: An Intimate Geography*. New York: Anchor Books, 2000.

Ayzad, *BDSM: Guida per esploratori dell'erotismo estremo*. Rome: Castelvecchi Editore, 2004.

Berthoz, Alain. *Le sense du mouvement*. Paris: Editions Odile Jacob, 2008.

Bishop, Clifford. *Sex and Spirit*. New York: Time-Life Editions, 1996.

Bodansky, Steve, and Vera Bodansky. *Extended Massive Orgasm: How You Can Give and Receive Intense Sexual Pleasure*. London: Vermilion, 2000.

Brame, Gloria G., Willam D. Brame and Jon Jacobs. *Different Loving: The World of Sexual Dominance and Submission*. New York: Villard, 1996.

Bullough, Bonnie, and Vern Bullough. *Women and Prostitution: A Social History*, Buffalo, N.Y.: Prometheus Press, 1987.

Caballo Santamaria, F., and R. Nesters. "Female Ejaculation: Myths and Reality." Paper presented at the 13th Congress of Sexology, Barcelona, Spain, August 29, 1997.

Calais-Geramin, Blandine. *Le périnée féminin et l'accouchement*. France: Editions Désiris, 2000.

Chalker, Rebecca. *The Clitoral Truth: The Secret World at Your Fingertips*. New York: Seven Stories Press, 2000.

Chapsal, Madeleine. *Conversations impudiques*. Paris: Editions Pauvert, 2002.

Chia, Mantak, and Douglas Abrams. *The Multi-Orgasmic Man: Sexual Secrets Every Man Should Know*. San Francisco: HarperOne, 1997.

Chia, Mantak, and Michael Wynn. *Taoist Secrets of Love*. New York: Aurora Press, 1985.

Comfort, Alex. *The Joy of Sex*. London: Mitchell Beazley, 2002.

Crompton, Louis. *Homosexuality and Civilization*. Cambridge, MA: Harvard University Press, 2003

Deguillon, Pierre-Louis. *Giochi erotici di società*. Milan: Sugarco edizioni, 1985.

De La Croix, Arnaud. *L'érotisme au Moyen Age*, Paris: Editions Tallandier, 2003.

Desikachar, T. K. V. *The Heart of Yoga: Developing a Personal Practice*. Rochester, VT: Inner Traditions, 1995. Italian translation *Il Cuore dello Yoga*. Rome: Casa edititrice Astrolabio-Ubaldini Editore, 1997.

Dodson, Betty. *Orgasms for Two*. New York: Harmony Books, 2002.

———. *Viva la Vulva: Women's Sex Organs Revealed*. Betty Dodson, 1998.

Dover, K. J. *Greek Homosexuality*. Cambridge, MA: Harvard University Press, 1989.

Douglas, Nik, and Penny Slinger. *Sexual Secrets: The Alchemy of Ecstasy*. Rochester, VT: Destiny Books, 1979.

Flaumenbaum, Dr. Danièle. *Femme désirée femme désirante*. Paris: Editions Payot, 2006.

Foer, Jonathan Safran. *Eating Animals*. London: Penguin Books, 2010.

Forberg, F. K. *Manuel d'erotologie classique*. Paris: Editions La Musardine, 1996.

Foucault, Michel. *Histoire de la sexualité, vol. 1: La Volonté de Savoir*; *2: L'usage des Plaisirs*; *3: Le Soucis de Soi*. Paris: Editions Gallimard, Paris, 2004.

Friedman, David M. *A Mind of Its Own: How Your Brain Distorts and Deceives*. London: Penguin Books, 2003.

Freud, Sigmund. *Three Essays on the Theory of Sexuality*. Edited and translated by James Strachey. New York: Basic Books, 2000.

———. *Sexuality and the Psychology of Love*. New York: Collier Books, 1963.

———. *Totem and Taboo*. Mineola, NY: Dover Thrift Editions, 1998.

Frobrose, Gabrielle, and Dr. Rolf Frobose. *Lust and Love: Is It More than Chemistry?* London: Royal Society of Chemistry Publishing, 2006.

Galimberti, Umberto. *I vizi capitali e i nuovi vizi*. Milan: Giangiacomo Feltrinelli Editore, 2004.

———. *Le cose dell'amore*. Milan: Giangiacomo Feltrinelli Editore, 2005.

———. *Il corpo*, Milan: Giangiacomo Feltrinelli Editore, 2003.

Godard, Odile. *La cuisine d'amour*. Paris: Editions Babel actes Sud, 1985.

Godson, Suzi. *The Body Bible*. London: Penguin Books, 2004.

Goleman, Daniel. *Emotional Intelligence: Why It Can Matter More than I.Q.* New York: Bantam Books, 2006.

Gray, John. *Men Are from Mars, Women Are from Venus: A Practical Guide for Improving Communication and Getting What You Want in Your Relationships*. London: Thorson, 1993.

Haich, Elisabeth. *Sexuelle Kraft und Yoga*. Hammelburg, Germany: Drei Eichen Verlag, 1973. French translation *Force sexuelle et yoga*. Lausanne, Switzerland: Editions Randin, 2001.

Hite, Shere. *The New Hite Report*. London: Hamlyn Publishing, 2002. French translation *Le nouveau rapport Hite*. Paris: Editions J'ai lu, 2002.

Hooper, Anne. *Massage erotique*, Paris: Editions contre-dires, 2005.

Jodorowsky, Alejandro. *La Danza de la Realidad*. Madrid: Siruela, 2001. Italian translation *La danza della realtà*. Milan, Italy: Giangiacomo Feltrinelli Editore, 2006.

————. *Psicomagia: Una terapia panica*. Milan: Giangiacomo Feltrinelli Editore, 2005.

Kakuro, Okakura. *Le petit livre du thé*. Translated by Gabriel Mourey. Paris: André Delpeuch Editeur, 1927.

Kaplan, Helen Singer. *Nuove terapie sessuali*. Milan: Bompiani Editions, 1982.

Ladas, Alice Kahn, and Beverly Whipple and John Perry. *The G Spot and Other Discoveries about Human Sexuality*. New York: Holt, Rinehart and Winston, 1982.

Leed, Cristina *Storia dell'amore libero*. Milan: Società Editoriale Attualità, 1967.

Leonelli, Elisabetta Leslie. *Al di la' delle labra*. Milan: Rizzoli Editions, 1983.

Levy, Ariel. *Female Chauvinist Pigs: Women and the Rise of Raunch Culture*. New York: Free Press, 2005.

Levy, Howard, and Ishihara Akira. *Il tao del sesso*. Milan: Xenia Edizioni, 1999.

Mac Orlan, Pierre. *Petite dactylo et autres textes de flagellation*. Paris: La Musardine Editions, 2005.

Masters, William H., and Virginia E. Johnson. *The Pleasure Bond*. New York: Bantam Books, 1974.

Masters, William H., and Virginia E. Johnson and Robert C. Kolodny. *Crisis: Heterosexual Behavior in the Age of AIDS*. New York: Grove Press, 1988.

Midori, *The Seductive Art of Japanese Bondage*. Emeryville, CA: Greenery Press, 2001.

Morin, Jack. *Anal Pleasure and Health*. San Francisco: Down There Press, 1998.

Morris, Desmond. *The Naked Ape*. London: Vintage Books, 1994.

Norwood, Robin. *Women Who Love Too Much*. London: Arrow Books, 2009.

Ovid. *L'art d'aimer*. Translation by d'Henri Bornecque. Paris: Editions Folio, 2004.

Paglia Camille, *Sexual Personae: Art and Decadence from Nefertiti to Emily Dickinson*. New York: Vintage Books, 1991.

Panati, Charles. *Sexy Origins and Intimate Things: The Rites and Rituals of Straights, Gays, Bis, Drags, Trans, Virgins, and Others*. London: Penguin Books, 1998.

Pasini, Willy. *Il cibo e l'amore*. Milan: Arnoldo Mondadori Editore, 1994.

————. *La vita a due: La scoppia a venti, quaranta e sessant' anni*. Milan: Arnoldo Mondadori Editore, 2007. French translation *Le couple amoureux*. Paris: Editions Odile Jacob, 2008.

Pasolini, P. Paolino. *Scritti corsari*. Milan: Garzanti Libri, 2005.

Perel, Esther. *Mating in Captivity: Sex, Lies, and Domestic Bliss*. New York: HarperCollins Publishers, 2006.

Piazza, Dalia, and Antonio Maglio. *Massaggio zonale del piede e della mano*. Milan: Giunti Demetra, 1999.

Pierri, Renato. *Sesso, diavolo e santità*. Rome: Coniglio Editore, 2007.

Plato, *The Symposium*. Translated by Walter Hamilton. London: Penguin Books, 1981.

Ramacharaka, Yogi. *Hatha Yoga*. Rome: Napoleone Editore, 1971.

Reinisch, June M. *The Kinsey Institute New Report on Sex*. New York: St. Martin's Press, 1991.

Rodenburg, Patsy. *The Second Circle: How to Use Positive Energy for Success in Every Situation*. London: W.W. Norton & Company, 2008.

Rubio-Casillas, A., and E. A. Jannini, MD. "New Insights from One Case of Female Ejaculation," *The Journal of Sexual Medicine* 8, no. 12 (December 2011): 3500–3504.

Sundahl, Deborah. *Female Ejaculation and the G-spot*. Alameda, CA: Hunter House, 2003.

Rumi. *The Book of Love: Poems of Ecstasy and Longing*. Translated and commentary by Coleman Barks. New York: HarperCollins, 2003.

Satyananda, Paramahamsa. *Asana Pranayama Mudra Bandha*. Milan: Edizioni Satyananda Ashram, 1997.

Sellers, Terence. *The Correct Sadist*. Philadelphia, PA: Temple Press, 1992.

Sevely, Josephine Lowndes. *Eve's Secrets: A New Theory of Female Sexuality*. New York: Random House, 1987.

Sevely, Josephine Lowndes, and J. W. Bennett. "Concerning Female Ejaculation and the Female Prostate," *Journal of Sex* 14 (1978): 1–20.

Sos, Dr. Paul. *La gym de l'Amour*. Paris: Presse du Chatelet, 1997.

Spencer, Colin. *Homosexuality: A History*. London: Fourth Estate, Ltd. 1995. French translation *Histoire de L'homosexualité*. Paris: Edition Pocket, 2005.

Tannahill, Reay. *Sex in History*. London: Abacus, 1996.

Thirleby, Ashley. *Tantra: The Key to Sexual Power*. London: Jaico Publishing House, 2006.

Travris, Carol. *The Mismeasure of Woman: Why Women Are Not the Better Sex, the Inferior Sex, or the Opposite Sex*. New York: Touchstone/Simon & 1993.

Van Lysebeth, André. *Pranayama la dynamique du Souffle*. Paris: Flammarion, 1971.

Vatsyayana. *Il kamasutra illustrato (Ananga Ranga: Il Giardino Profumato)* Translation by Virginia Teodori. Rome: Gruppo Editoriale L'Espresso, 2002.

Vidal, Gore. *Sexually Speaking: Collected Sex Writings*. San Francisco: Clies Press, 1999.

West, Mae. *On Sex, Health & ESP*. London: W. H. Allen, 1975.

Yhuel, Isabelle. *Les femmes et leur plaisir*. Paris: JC Lattès, 2001.

Zander, Rosamund Stone, and Benjamin Zander. *The Art of Possibility: Transforming Professional and Personal Life*. New York: Penguin Group, 2002.

ACKNOWLEDGMENTS

———o———

THE BOUDOIR BIBLE grew out of a miniature guide that I provided with my jewelry designs and the preparatory notes that I took before teaching my Sexual Skills salons. As the Paradise Found collection grew, the miniature guide no longer sufficed, and as my salons evolved, I realized that the only way to reach a wider public was to write a book. I would like to thank my ex-husband, Barnaba Fornasetti, for his ongoing support and friendship; Malaika King Albrecht, poet and my lifelong friend, for helping me to structure the first version of the text with her invaluable insight; and Terence Sellers, for helping me proof the second version of the text. Many thanks go to Charles Miers, the publisher of Rizzoli and my editor, Dung Ngo, who believed in *The Boudoir Bible* and made sure it saw the light of day. Dung, I thank you, as well, for bringing Elizabeth Smith on board; with her magic word wand, open mind, and good sense of humor, the manuscript came to fruition. Richard Pandiscio, my book designer and Francois Berthoud, my illustrator, thank you for both for injecting visual vitality into every page of *The Boudoir Bible*.

I would also like to thank all of the couples and individuals who have sought out my support and guidance during their sexual journeys, including those who have participated in my Sexual Skills salons in the U.K., France, North America, and Italy: you have my deepest gratitude.

I would also like to thank all of my ceremonial partners and the present love of my life, as well as each and every one of my friends for their love, patience, trust, and support. I would never have managed to finish this work without the sweet distractions that we share. Rhett Butler, Nigel Coates, Eric Treiber, Manuel Aymonier, Zsolt Rendetzki, Olivier Zahm, Claire Czajkowska, Danica Lepen, Yasmin Gross, Marianne Costa, Marie-France Boutet, and Al, thank you for helping me push things along when the going got really tough. Aimee Mullins, my dear, dear friend, our epic discussions about the limits of categories and the power of differences helped me challenge and fine-tune my ideas. There are no words with which to express my gratitude for all of your precious input.

Finally, I would like to thank my father, for teaching me the art of possibility; and my mother, who was also my biggest fan, for championing my mission to empower men and women to enjoy and experience greater sexual pleasure.

First published in the United States of America in 2013 by
Rizzoli International Publications
300 Park Avenue South
New York, NY 10010
www.rizzoliusa.com

ISBN-13: 978-0-8478-4016-8
Library of Congress Control Number: 2012947521

Editor: Dung Ngo
Copy Editor: Elizabeth Smith

Creative Direction: Richard Pandiscio
Design: William Loccisano and Tim Lahan / Pandiscio Co.

Printed and bound in the China

2019 2020 2021 2022 2023 / 10 9 8 7 6 5 4